AF556907

Fine Needle Aspiration of Bone Tumours

Monographs in Clinical Cytology

Vol. 19

Series Editor

Svante R. Orell Kent Town

Fine Needle Aspiration of Bone Tumours

The Clinical, Radiological, Cytological Approach

Måns Åkerman Lund
Henryk A. Domanski Lund
Kjell Jonsson Lund

88 figures, 61 in color, and 10 tables, 2010

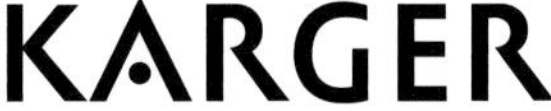

Basel · Freiburg · Paris · London · New York · Bangalore · Bangkok · Shanghai · Singapore · Tokyo · Sydney

Monographs in Clinical Cytology

Dr. Måns Åkerman
Department of Pathology and Cytology
University Hospital
SE-221 85 Lund (Sweden)

Dr. Kjell Jonsson
Department of Radiology
University Hospital
SE-221 85 Lund (Sweden)

Dr. Henryk A. Domanski
Department of Pathology and Cytology
University Hospital
SE-221 85 Lund (Sweden)

Library of Congress Cataloging-in-Publication Data

Åkerman, Måns.
Fine needle aspiration of bone tumours : the clinical, radiological, cytological approach / Måns Åkerman, Henryk A. Domanski, Kjell Jonsson.
p. ; cm. -- (Monographs in clinical cytology, ISSN 0077-0809 ; v. 19)
Includes bibliographical references and index.
ISBN 978-3-8055-9214-7 (hard cover : alk. paper)
1. Bones--Tumors--Diagnosis. 2. Bones--Radiography. 3. Cytodiagnosis. I. Domanski, Henryk A. II. Jonsson, Kjell, Dr. III. Title.
[DNLM: 1. Bone Neoplasms--diagnosis. 2. Bone Neoplasms--radiography. 3. Biopsy, Fine-Needle--methods. 4. Cytological Techniques--methods. W1 MO567KF v.19 2010 / WE 258 A314f 2010]
RC280.B6A37 2010
616.99'471075--dc22

2009032398

Bibliographic Indices. This publication is listed in bibliographic services, including Current Contents®.

www.karger.com
Printed in Switzerland on acid-free and non-aging paper (ISO 9706) by Reinhardt Druck, Basel
ISSN 0077–0809
ISBN 978–3–8055–9214–7
e-ISBN 978–3–8055–9215–4

Contents

Preface

At the beginning of the 1960s Nils Stormby, at that time head of the recently founded Cytodiagnostic Laboratory, introduced fine needle aspiration (FNA) and cytodiagnosis as the primary diagnostic modality in cases of bone tumours/lesions in Lund, Sweden. When the Musculoskeletal Tumour Centre was created at the University Hospital, FNA became the primary diagnostic method for bone tumours/lesions in patients referred to the centre. From the beginning, the centre's orthopaedic surgeons and radiologists established a close working relationship, and their experience clearly demonstrated the importance of the clinical, radiological and cytological approach to diagnosis. In 1973, the diagnostic outcome of the first 94 cases, which were investigated between 1966 and 1969, was presented and discussed [1].

Although it has been strongly recommended that patients with suspected bone tumours/lesions should be referred to multidisciplinary centres for primary diagnosis and treatment, in practice this is not always the case, especially in patients with suspected metastatic deposits. The purpose of this book is to emphasize the value of the combined diagnostic approach, and to facilitate the cytological evaluation of FNA smears from hard tissue lesions. We also suggest criteria for histotype diagnosis based on the combined evaluation of clinical and radiographic data and cytologic features. Our main aim is to thoroughly describe and illustrate the most common entities. A number of primary bone tumours/ lesions, benign as well as malignant, are very rare and their cytologic features have been described only incompletely, if at all.

The use of adjunctive diagnostic methods is also described, discussed and illustrated. The selection of entities described and illustrated are based mainly on experiences with patients referred to the Musculoskeletal Centre over a 35-year period. Case reports and illustrations are culled from cases in the files of the Department of Pathology and Cytology, Lund University Hospital, which now comprise smears from approximately 1,000 hard tissue tumours/ lesions dated between 1966 and 2006.

Acknowledgements

The authors are grateful for the help given by Dr. Svante Orell, Adelaide, Australia. Dr. Orell is the scientific editor for the series *Monographs in Clinical Cytology* and his comments on the text and revisions of the language have been of great help. We also thank Dr. Walter Ryd, Head of the Division of Cytology, Department of Pathology, Sahlgren's Hospital, Gothenburg, Sweden, for letting us use illustrations of cases of very rare bone tumours.

Måns Åkerman
Henryk A. Domanski
Kjell Jonsson
Lund

Chapter 1

Epidemiology of Bone Tumours

As primary bone tumours are relatively uncommon, it is difficult to assemble meaningful data with regard to their relative frequency and incidence.

An extensive investigation of the data on 2,627 cases collected between 1973 and 1987 from 9 geographical areas in the United States showed that primary bone sarcomas constituted only 0.2% of all malignant tumors (table 1) [2]. The incidence rate was 0.8/100,000, and showed no tendency to change during the time period under study.

According to the Swedish National Cancer Registry 2004, the incidence rate per 100,000 inhabitants was 0.6 for chondrosarcoma, 0.42 for osteosarcoma and 0.29 for Ewing's sarcoma.

The relative frequencies are reported below exclude lymphohaematopoetic tumours. In the above investigation, osteosarcoma was the most frequent primary bone sarcoma, followed by chondrosarcoma, Ewing's sarcoma and chordoma. There were only 4 cases of adamantinoma among the 2,627 cases studied.

One major monograph on bone tumors [3] reviewed 4,138 malignant primary bone tumours. In this series osteosarcoma was the most frequent tumour, followed by chondrosarcoma, Ewing's sarcoma and chordoma. Twenty-three adamantinomas were diagnosed among the cases studied. There were 2,028 benign tumours. The 5 most common benign tumours were osteochondroma, giant cell tumour, chondroma, osteid osteoma and metaphyseal fibrous defect.

Table 1. Frequency of 2,627 primary malignant bone tumours [2]

Tumour type	Frequency	%
Osteosarcoma	922	35
Chondrosarcoma	677	26
Ewing's sarcoma	420	16
Chordoma	221	8
Malignant fibrous histiocytoma	78	3
Angiosarcoma	36	1
Adamantinoma	4	0.2

Lymphohaematopoetic tumours are excluded from the data.

Table 2. Summary of distribution of malignant bone tumours by histologic type and patient age [3]

Tumour	Decade								%	Total n
	1	2	3	4	5	6	7	8		
Osteosarcoma		601	228						65	1,274
Chondrosarcoma					110	132			44	545
Ewing's sarcoma	72	231							75	402
Chordoma						69	54		47	262

Lymphohaematopoetic tumours are excluded from the data.

Table 3. Summary and distribution of benign bone tumours by histological type and patient age [3]

Tumour	Decade								%	Total n
	1	2	3	4	5	6	7	8		
Osteochondroma/ chondroma		420	180						62	972
Giant cell			165	99					62	425
Chondroblastoma		43	11						68	79
Osteid osteoma		130	56						76	245
Osteoblastoma		28	20						76	63
Chondromyx.fibr		10	12						56	39

The distribution of malignant and benign bone tumours by histological type and by age of patient is summarized in tables 2 and 3, respectively. From the tables it is obvious that the majority of benign bone tumours, osteosarcoma and Ewing's sarcoma, are found in patients between 20 and 40 years of age, while chondrosarcoma and chordoma occur most frequently after the age of 50 years.

It is also obvious that a number of benign bone tumours are relatively infrequent, which is of importance in defining diagnostic cytological criteria.

Chapter 2

Radiological Investigation of Bone Tumours

Patients with bone tumours are usually motivated to seek medical consultation after noticing some type of symptom, such as pain, a palpable tumour or reduced functing of a joint or extremity.

The first radiological investigation is usually plain radiography of the symptomatic site. In most instances there is some type of change in the texture of the involved bone. There may be bone destruction or a periosteal reaction at the involved site. The most important radiographic observation is to recognize that there is a bony change present. Other modalities must be used to further evaluate the extent of the lesion, any soft tissue component or spread. The image on plain radiography may appear typical for a certain histological type of tumour, but often the first impression is wrong as regards tumour typing. The saying 'anything can look like anything' is definitely true for the radiological appearance of bone tumours.

Tumour Type and Radiological Appearance

Types of bone tumour are considered to correspond to various radiological findings. Three different patterns can be distinguished, which are arranged below by increasing generally assumed aggressiveness.

- Geographic lesion. A well-demarcated destruction with or without a thin sclerotic margin (fig. 1a).
- Moth-eaten lesion. A poorly demarcated lesion of the bone marrow (fig. 1b).
- Permeative lesion. A poorly demarcated lesion of the bone marrow and the cortical bone (fig. 1c).

The geographic, well-demarcated lesion is considered to be a slowly growing tumour, in most cases a benign cystic lesion. However, there are exceptions, and solitary plasmocytoma and metastatic tumours may have a geographic growth pattern.

More aggressive malignant tumours, such as Ewing's sarcoma, osteosarcoma and chondrosarcoma usually show a moth-eaten or permeative pattern. It is, however, to be remembered that even osteomyelitis may show a very aggressive appearance and can not be excluded on the basis of radiological findings.

There are some characteristic findings that can further categorise a lesion, which are outlined below.

Tumour Matrix Calcifications

These may be a characteristic sign of some lesions. Speckled calcifications are often the main diagnostic clue to a correct diagnosis in chondromatous tumours. The appearance of the calcifications does not indicate whether the lesion is malignant or benign. For example, the differential diagnosis of a lesion with bone marrow calcifications includes a bone infarct. An osteosarcoma may be mainly sclerotic (i.e. with calcified matrix), it may be mixed osteolytic and sclerotic, or it may be mainly lytic. The pattern does not correlate with the degree of malignancy or clinical behaviour. However, speckled calcifications in a permeative lesion indicate a chondrosarcoma. Homogenous calcifications may be seen in osteosarcoma and are a characteristic of parosteal osteosarcoma.

Periosteal Reaction

This is an important feature in tumour diagnosis. The periosteal reaction may have various appearances, such as cortical thickening, onion-peel like, spicula formation and Codman's triangle. Onion-peel appearance and spicula formation are obvious and are immediately indicative of malignancy, while Codman's triangle may be subtle and easily overlooked. This periosteal reaction is a result of elevation of the periosteum due to a soft tissue component adjacent to the triangular calcification, which does not

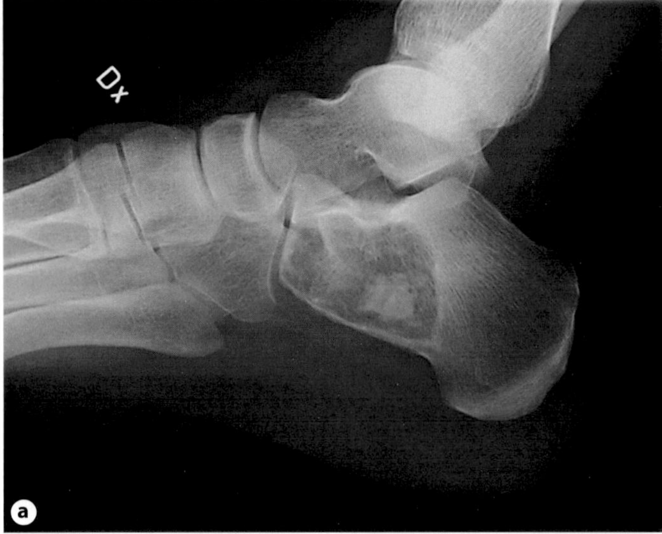

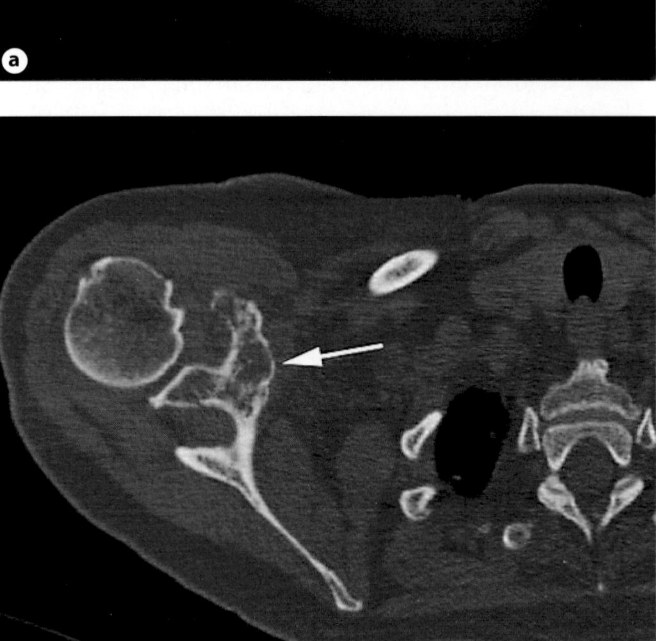

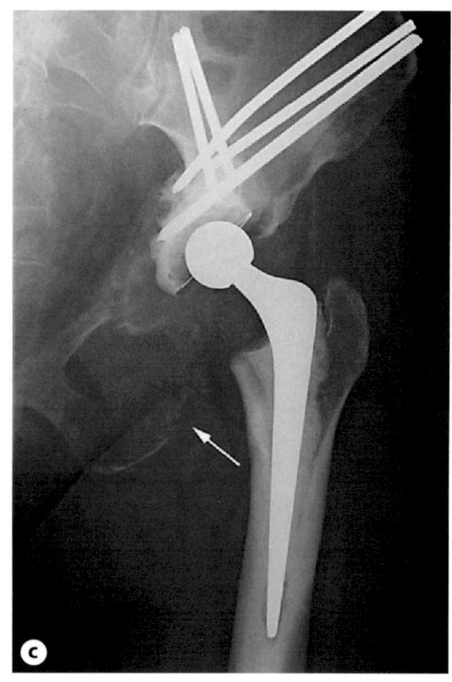

Fig. 1. a Geographic lesion. Aneurysmal bone cyst of the calcaneus with well defined borders. **b** Moth-eaten tumour type. Lesion of the scapula of unknown nature. CT of the scapula, where the lesion is easily visible (arrow). **c** Permeative tumour growth. The patient had metastatic breast cancer to the ischium and the pubic bone.

contain tumour tissue but is only a reaction to the elevation of the periosteum. The presence and type of a periosteal reaction does not provide any clue to the histological type of tumour.

Soft Tissue Component

A soft tissue component is indicative of a malignant tumour, but does not in itself give any clues to the type of tumour. Soft tissue extensions are most common in Ewing's sarcoma and osteosarcoma, but may also be present in chondrosarcoma.

Tumour Position

Where a tumour is positioned in the long bones may be a diagnostic sign.

Mainly Involving the Epiphysis. Tumour growth in the epiphysis is rare, and the most common type of lesion is chondroblastoma. When such a lesion contains small calcifications the diagnosis is clear.

Giant cell tumours are located eccentrically in the metaphysis-epiphysis, often grow close to the subchondral area of a joint (most often around the knee) and display a geographic growth pattern.

Metaphysis. The metaphysis is the most common site for tumours. This is probably due to the fast turnover of growing cells adjacent to the growth plate. Osteosarcoma typically arises in the metaphyseal region.

Diaphyseal. A diaphyseal location is very common in Ewing's sarcoma.

The tumour position in the long bones may be further defined. Benign cysts, which are well demarcated and show a geographic growth pattern, are usually located centrally in the metaphysis. Intracortical tumours are most often metastatic. Parosteal lesions arise from the cortical bone with extension outside the bone in a mushroom pattern. The tumour grows parallel to the cortical bone and there is a cleft between the tumour mass and the cortical bone, best visualized on a CT scan. Destructive lesions of the sacrum may be extensive, with a soft tissue component ventrally as well as dorsally. The most commonly suggested diagnosis is chordoma, but the same radiological appearance may be seen in giant cell tumours or metastases in the sacrum. In such cases patient age is of importance. In a 60-year-old male the most likely diagnosis is metastasis or chordoma, while in a 20-year-old female the most probable diagnosis is a giant cell tumour.

Other Investigations

The various methods of investigation to define a bone lesion complement each other.

Magnetic Resonance Imaging

Radiological findings are usually more characteristic than findings on MRI, which is a mandatory modality for investigation of a known or suspected tumour. The main advantage of MRI is its ability to define the extent of a tumour in relation to the bone marrow, cortical destruction and soft tissue extension. When tumours in the long bones are evaluated with MRI, the whole of that bone must be examined in order to detect so-called skip lesions (intramedullary metastases in the same bone). In cystic lesions, MRI may demonstrate several compartments with fluid levels typically indicating an aneurysmal bone cyst or, rarely, an osteosarcoma.

Computed Tomography

CT is very sensitive to show or rule out even subtle bone destruction. CT is also the method of choice to detect tumour calcifications, which are poorly diagnosed with MRI. However, the full size of a bone marrow extension is poorly demonstrated with CT. Fluid levels can be seen easily on CT.

The modern multislice CT technique has made it possible to make reconstructions in all orthogonal planes, and to use CT as an alternative to MRI for the evaluation of soft tissue extension, especially after the infusion of intravenous contrast medium.

Ultrasonography

Ultrasonography is rarely used in bone tumour investigations. A soft tissue component is easily diagnosed, and cortical destruction may be visible.

Scintigraphy

Bone scintigraphy is a good method to evaluate metastases, either from an unknown primary tumour or from a bone tumour. It is a sensitive, but non-specific, method. As fractures and inflammatory and degenerative bone reactions may simulate metastases, the scintigraphy should be evaluated in combination with radiographic examinations.

Positron Emisson Tomography

PET and CT-PET are the latest diagnostic developments in bone tumour diagnosis. Most commonly, short-lived isotopes are incorporated in a metabolic substance, and increases in metabolic activity indicate the degree of malignancy. This applies both to soft tissue tumours, bone tumours and inflammatory conditions. In combination with CT it is easy to locate exactly the site of activity.

As has been emphasized, radiological findings are often non-specific, and a tissue diagnosis is necessary to supplement the radiological evaluation.

Fine Needle Aspiration Cytology

This can be easily be performed when guided by the radiological findings. In cases of clear-cut bone destruction, the needling can be performed with fluoroscopic guidance. CT-guided aspiration biopsy should be the method of choice for deep lesions. Another advantage with CT is that the full extent of the tumour can be evaluated and the needle directed to various parts of large tumours.

In open MRI systems, aspiration biopsy can be performed using special non-ferromagnetic needles.

Conclusion

The radiological investigation includes several modalities – plain radiography, ultrasonography, MRI, CT, scintigraphy and PET – which are all important in the evaluation of a bone tumours. The choice of method(s) may differ from institution to institution, depending on the equipment available and the experience of the radiologists.

The most important task for the radiologist is to evaluate the extent of the tumour, not the tissue diagnosis, even if findings may indicate a certain histotype. In this aspect the cooperation between radiologist and cytopathologist is mandatory. The radiological findings may confirm the tissue diagnosis, but must be re-evaluated in cases of discordance between the results from radiological imaging and tissue analyses.

Chapter 3

Morphological Diagnosis of Bone Tumours

Biopsies

Open Biopsy

Open biopsy and histopathological assessment of tissue samples has for many years been considered to be the method of choice to diagnose bone tumours/lesions. However, open biopsy has a number of disadvantages: the patient must be hospitalized, general anaesthesia is often required, the biopsy may breach compartments and there is a risk of haematoma and infection.

Percutaneous Biopsy

Methods for percutaneous sampling, such as core needle biopsy (CNB) and drill biopsy, have during recent years emerged as important diagnostic substitutes for open biopsy. Percutaneous sampling can be performed in outpatient clinics, most often with local rather than general anaesthesia.

The results from 4 recent investigations, comprising 470 patients, are summarized in table 4 [4–7].

Fine Needle Aspiration Cytology

Fine needle aspiration cytology (FNAC) has been used for many years in the diagnosis of bone tumours/lesions. As early as 1931, Coley et al. [8] applied this sampling method, and since then several large series of cases have been published [1, 9–18].

Compared to open biopsy, both FNAC and CNB have the advantages of being performed under ambulatory conditions without the need for hospitalization or, in the majority of cases, general anaesthesia.

Compared to CNB, FNAC is less traumatic, has a lower frequency of complications and, in most cases, the cytomorphology of the aspirated material is superior to that in a CNB. Using aspiration it is possible to sample sufficient material for immunocytochemical evaluation, molecular genetic analyses and other adjunctive diagnostic methods by FNA. The aspirated material is, however, not always sufficient for ancillary techniques. The advantages of CNB compared to FNA are 2-fold: (1) it is usually possible to study the tissue architecture of the tumour, and (2) in most cases the sampled material is sufficient for routine microscopic examination as well as for various ancillary techniques.

FNAC Procedure

Due to their often destructive growth and frequent soft tissue extension, the majority of primary malignant bone tumours are suitable targets for sampling using thin needles of 23–21 gauge (0.6–0.8 mm). It is usually difficult or impossible to penetrate intact cortical bone with these thin needles, but destroyed or 'moth-eaten' cortical bone can be penetrated fairly easily. When the cortex is intact, some investigators advocate using an 18-gauge (1.1 mm) needle to penetrate the cortical bone and thereafter insert a 23-gauge (0.6 mm) needle through the larger needle. Alternatively, the Bone Biopty instrument, a coaxial biopsy system with an eccentric drill, invented by Ahlström and Åström, may be used [19]. In such instances local anaesthesia is necessary, and in children perhaps even a short general anaesthesia.

In our institution we seldom use FNAC as a diagnostic procedure for intra-osseous lesions when the cortical bone in entirely intact.

Palpable bone tumours are most often successfully needled by the cytopathologist but non-palpable lesions are better needled with radiological guidance, either by a radiologist trained in the aspiration technique or jointly by the cytopathologist and the radiologist.

The equipment used for FNA of bone lesions is the same as for needling other sites. A syringe holder permitting

Table 4. CNB for bone tumours. A summary of diagnostic yield and accuracy according to 4 recent series

Authors	Cases n	Insufficient yield, %	Diagnostic accuracy, %[1]
Pramesh et al., 2001 [4]	136	11	97
Jelinek et al., 2002 [5]	110	not listed	88
Ossakov et al., 2003 [6]	135	not listed	87
Viellard et al., 2005 [7]	89	31	not listed

[1] Core vs. final diagnosis.

aspiration with one hand is essential. In most cases, 22-gauge (0.7 mm) needles are sufficient. The length of the needle depends on the location of the lesion. Needles with a stylet are recommended for deep-seated tumours/lesions. The stylet strengthens the needle and prevents the aspiration of cells from surrounding tissues. Close communication with the surgeon is important as she may wish to decide the point of needle insertion in palpable cases suspicious of malignancy. In cases of clinically suspected malignancy, the insertion point suggested by the surgeon is tattooed so that the needle track can be removed at surgery.

Staining Methods

Generally, the best diagnostic results are achieved by evaluating air-dried smears, stained with DiffQuick or May-Grünwald Giemsa (MGG), or ethanol-fixed smears, stained with hematoxylin and eosin (HE) or according to Papanicolau (Pap).

Wet-fixed smears are superior for evaluation of nuclear details such as nuclear membrane, chromatin texture and nucleoli, while background matrix and cytoplasmic details are better elucidated in air-dried material.

Ancillary Diagnostic Techniques

The interpretation of routinely stained smears is the basis for the cytological evaluation of bone tumours/lesions. For example, the presence of osteoid, visible in May-Grünwald-Giemsa-stained smears, is one important diagnostic criterion of osteosarcoma in a malignant aspirate [15]. However, ancillary diagnostics are indispensable to reach a reliable diagnosis in selected cases, especially those in which the treatment includes neoadjuvant therapy followed by surgery. Osteosarcoma and Ewing's sarcoma/primitive neuroectodermal tumour (PNET) are examples of tumours in which the cytological diagnosis in all aspects must be fully equivalent to a histopathological diagnosis based on a tissue sample.

Essentially, the same special diagnostic procedures applied to tissue samples are applicable on fine needle aspirates. The current ancillary methods are cytochemistry, immunocytochemistry, DNA ploidy analysis, flow cytometric immunophenotyping in lymphohaematological lesions, cytogenetic and molecular genetic investigations and to some extent electron microscopic examination.

Various preparation methods are in use for cytochemical and immunocytochemical stainings.

Direct Smears

Direct smears can be difficult to evaluate due to the cellular trauma inherent in the technique. When nuclei are stripped of their cytoplasm it is impossible to assess the result of cytochemical staining and immunostaining with cytoplasmic antibodies, while direct smears, according to our experience, function well with nuclear antibodies.

Cytospin Preparations

Cytospin preparations are probably the most commonly used technique for cytochemical and immunocytochemical stainings. It is evident that the efficacy in using cytospin preparations varies from laboratory to laboratory. In our experience, when the antibody expression is focal in a tumour sample, false negative results are not unusual in cytospin preparations.

Cell Block Preparation from Formalin-Fixed and Paraffin-Embedded Aspirates

Cell-block preparations are, when successful, comparable to a mini-biopsy and are suitable for all antibodies used in the histopathological evaluation of tumours. It is easy to compare the staining results in a cell block with a subsequent biopsy or surgical specimens. Furthermore, a routinely stained cell block might give information on tumour architecture. Our experience is that cell-block preparations are better vehicles for immunocytochemistry than cytospin preparations.

Liquid-Based Cytology: ThinPrep

ThinPrep has emerged as a new and common technique to prepare FNA samples for immunostaining. Among the advantages of ThinPrep are a clean background, a monolayer

Table 5. Useful antibodies in the diagnosis of primary bone tumours/lesions

Tumour/lesion	Antibody panel	Notes
Chondrosarcoma	S-100 protein	strong staining in low-grade malignant tumours; weak staining in high-grade malignant tumours
Chordoma	S-100 protein, cytokeratin	double staining of tumour cells
Ewing family of tumours	CD99, FLI-1	membrane staining for CD99; nuclear staining for FLI-1
Langerhan cell histiocytosis	S-100 protein, CD1	CD1 more specific than S-100 protein
Osteosarcoma	osteocalcin, osteonectin	see [39, 40]
Primary non-Hodgkin lymphoma		
Diffuse large B-cell lymphoma	CD20, CD3, BCL-6	
Precursor lymphoma	CD3, CD79A, CD10, TdT	
Anaplastic large-cell lymphoma	CD30, EMA, Alk-1, CD2, CD3, CD4	
Plasmocytoma	CD138, kappa/lambda	

of cells and that preparations may be saved unstained for further use. Our experience with immunostaining of ThinPrep prepared from fine needle aspirates of bone tumours has so far been promising, but further experience with various antibodies is needed before a definitive opinion of its value can be formed.

Cytochemistry

Alkaline phosphatase (ALP) staining is useful in the demonstration of osteoblastic differentiation of tumour cells in aspirates from osteosarcoma, as tumour cells from all subtypes of osteosarcoma contain abundant cytoplasmic ALP. Strong ALP positivity confirms the osteosarcoma diagnosis and helps to distinguish metastatic carcinoma or malignant melanoma and primary anaplastic large-cell lymphoma of bone from high-grade osteosarcoma. ALP staining in the cytological evaluation of osteosarcoma has been underestimated in previous reports of FNA-diagnosis of osteosarcoma. In our series of 59 primary osteosarcoma examined by FNA, strong cytoplasmic ALP-positivity could be demonstrated in all 30 cases in which this method was applied [15]. We currently use unstained air-dried slides for ALP-staining tumour cells in pleomorphic sarcoma of the malignant fibrous histiocytoma. However, the ALP staining in malignant fibrous histiocytoma is predominantly localized in the spindly cells, whereas in our cases nearly all tumour cells in osteosarcoma showed strong positivity. Other examples of the diagnostic use of cytochemistry is Periodic acid-Schiff staining to demonstrate cytoplasmic glycogen in clear-cell chondrosarcoma.

Immunocytochemistry

Immunocytochemical staining is particularly useful in the typing of the small-cell malignant tumours in bone aspirates, and in the distinction of metastatic carcinoma, melanoma metastases and primary anaplastic large-cell lymphoma from osteosarcoma.

Other examples are the important use of immunostaining in the definitive diagnosis of Langerhans cell histiocytosis and in the subtyping of malignant lymphoma.

In table 5 useful antibodies are presented.

Flow Cytometric Immunophenotyping

For many years we have used flow cytometric immunophenotyping as a diagnostic complement in case of suspected non-Hodgin lymphoma, primary in-bone and secondary deposits. Above all, the immunophenotyping is important in the differential diagnosis of indolent B-cell lymphoma and reactive lymphocytosis. Using a battery of antibodies it is also possible to define the lymphoma subtype.

DNA Ploidy Analysis

DNA ploidy analysis is, based on our experience, a valuable diagnostic complement in the diagnosis of osteosarcoma and in the differential diagnosis between enchondroma and chondrosarcoma. Conventional high-grade malignant osteosarcomas are usually non-diploid when tissue samples are investigated [20] as are most cases of grade II and III chondrosarcoma [21, 22]. We have had similar results with ploidy analysis of aspirates. We have found that aspirates are suitable for flow cytometric analysis as well for as static cytometry.

One advantage with static cytometry, performed on aspirative smears is that a routinely stained smear can be destained and then restained with a Feulgen staining.

In our experience, an unequivocal non-diploid histogram is strongly suggestive of malignancy in cases of suspected conventional osteosarcoma and chondrosarcoma.

Cytogenetic and Molecular Genetic Investigations

These techniques have, during recent years, emerged as very powerful diagnostic tools in the diagnosis of soft-tissue sarcoma. With regard to bone neoplasms, the main use of these techniques is in the diagnosis of Ewing's sarcoma/PNET. In our experience, and that of others, fine needle aspirates are less suitable for conventional karyotyping because the number of tumour cells obtained is often insufficient for tissue culture [23, 24]. Fine needle aspirates have proved very suitable for molecular genetic investigations such as RT-PCR and fluorescence in situ hybridization [25].

Electron Microscopic Examination

At present, electron microscopic examination as an adjunctive method has in part been replaced by immunocytochemistry and molecular genetic analyses. However, electron microscopy is still of importance in the diagnosis of certain entities, as in the demonstration of Birbeck's granules in Langerhans cell histiocytosis, of osteoid in case of osteosarcoma and in the differentiation of the small-cell malignant tumours such as Ewing's sarcoma/PNET and rhabdomyosarcoma.

Diagnosis of Bone Tumours/Lesions

Ideally, needle samples from the first pass should be stained immediately using DiffQuick or rapid HE or Pap, and checked to confirm that the material is sufficient and that the cells are interpretable. Immediate examination also allows the cytopathologist to broadly assess the type of lesion (chondromatous tumour, small cell tumour, suspicion of osteosarcoma or metastatic lesion, etc.) and to decide whether more

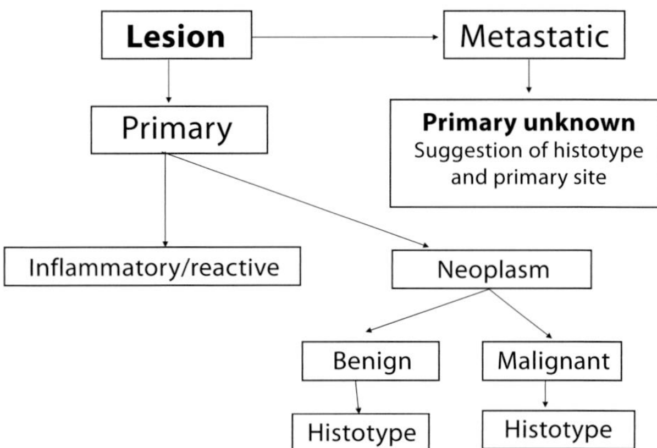

Fig. 2. Microscopic examination of an aspirate from a bone tumour/lesion. A summary of the diagnostic steps considered to reach the final diagnosis.

material is required and if ancillary techniques are likely to be needed to achieve a diagnosis.

As emphasized in Chapter 2, cooperation between orthopaedic surgeon, radiologist and cytologist is essential. The final diagnosis of an aspirate from a bone tumour/lesion should be the combined evaluation of clinical data, radiographic findings and the cytological examination. When patients are referred to an orthopaedic tumour centre where investigations are carried out by a multidisciplinary team, the collaboration between orthopaedic surgeon, radiologist and cytologist obviously results in a combination diagnosis. When this is not the case, it is mandatory that the cytologist has access to all available information on the radiographic findings (site, size and type of lesion) and that she correlates these with clinical data (age of the patient, patient history) and with the cytological features.

The importance of the radiological-cytological approach to the diagnosis has been clearly demonstrated by Söderlund et al. [18]. Out of 357 evaluable cases, there was compliance between radiology and cytology in 256 with a diagnostic error rate of 1%, while the error rate in the 101 non-compliant cases was 17%.

Classification of the Cytodiagnosis

The diagnostic steps towards the final diagnosis are summarized in figure 2.

A standardized reporting format benefits both the orthopaedic surgeon and the cytopathologist. Söderlund [26] proposed the use of 6 diagnostic categories: (1) sarcoma (histotype may or may not be specified); (2) benign tumour (histotype defined or not); (3) metastasis (or

Table 6. Standardized reporting of FNA-diagnosis of bone tumours (according to Soderlund [26] with minor modifications)

Sarcoma (histotype defined or not: sarcoma not otherwise specified)
Benign tumour (histotype defined or not: benign tumour not otherwise specified)
Metastasis (primary defined or descriptive diagnosis: adenocarcinoma, squamous cell carcinoma, etc.)
Lymphohaematologic malignancy (type defined or broad classification: malignant lymphoma, non-Hodgkin lymphoma, etc.)
Non-neoplastic lesion (infectious, reactive)
Non-diagnostic (benign vs. malignant; primary vs. metastasis)
Insufficient

Table 7. FNAC of bone tumours/lesions: number of cases with insufficient yield and accuracy

Authors	Cases n	Insufficient yield, %	False diagnosis (benign vs. malignant), %
Kreicsbergs et al., 1996 [12]	300	8	3.3
Bommer et al., 1997 [13]	450	14	2.2
Åkerman and Domanski, 1998 [15]	333	6	1.5
Jorda et al., 2000 [16]	314	31	13
Söderlund et al., 2004 [18]	370	3	5

Pertinent data are summarized from 5 recent series, comprising 1,767 patients.

lymphohaematological malignancies); (4) non-neoplastic lesions (infectious/reactive); (5) normal cells, and (6) non-diagnostic (insufficient material or non-diagnostic). In our opinion metastases should be separated from lymphohaematological malignancies. Our suggested reporting format is shown in table 6.

Examples of cytodiagnostic reports: primary bone sarcoma (radiology and cytology well compatible with osteosarcoma); primary benign bone tumour with numerous osteoclast-like giant cells (radiological findings typical for giant cell tumour).

Diagnostic Accuracy Bone Lesion FNA

Several reports of diagnostic accuracy with regard to benignity and malignancy have been published. The results of 5 large series comprising a total of almost 1,800 patients are summarized in table 7. The diagnostic accuracy regarding benign versus malignant was between 87 and 98% in these series.

It is also interesting to note that in 4 of these 5 studies, the material was insufficient for diagnosis only in 3–14% of cases. From table 7 it may be concluded that adequate sampling for microscopic evaluation of bone lesions is in no way inferior compared to FNA of parenchymatous organs or soft-tissue tumours.

Above all, the ability of FNA to correctly diagnose the histotype depends on compliance with the radiological diagnosis (combination diagnosis) and the use of ancillary diagnostic methods. A type-specific diagnosis is easier to achieve in malignant bone lesions than in benign bone tumours.

Pitfalls in Bone Tumour FNA

There are 3 important limitations to FNAC in the diagnosis of bone tumours.

(1) Inability to aspirate sufficient material for evaluation. The radiological features of a bone lesion often decide whether an aspiration succeeds or not. Important negative factors for a diagnostic aspirate are an intact cortex, sclerosis, heavy calcifications and purely intramedullary lesions.

(2) Sampling error. When tumours with a heterogeneous architecture are needled, the aspirated material might not correspond to the diagnostic tissue. An example of this pitfall is the aspiration of giant-cell-rich osteosarcoma when the smears are dominated by benign osteoclast-like cells.

(3) Poor or technically suboptimal material. Extensive necrosis or haemorrhage are limiting factors.

Misinterpretation of the material can also be a pitfall. There are several documented diagnostic difficulties, which shall be discussed in the following chapters. Definitive cytological criteria have not yet been established for relatively rare primary bone tumours, especially for some benign entities and for some histotypes. Well known diagnostic difficulties are enchondroma versus low-grade malignant chondrosarcoma, chondromyxoid fibroma versus chondrosarcoma, osteosarcoma in elderly patients and the histotype diagnosis in the heterogeneous group of benign bone tumours/lesions exhibiting numerous osteoclast-like giant cells in the smears.

Complications of Bone Tumour FNA

We have more than 30 years' experience of FNA in the primary diagnosis of bone tumours/lesions in patients referred to our musculoskeletal tumour centre, and in that time we have never experienced any severe complication. Patients have, at most, complained of brief pain at needling but we have never seen cases of infection or tumour cell seeding in the needle track.

Examples of severe complications documented in single cases are pneumothorax following needling of tumours in the ribs and neurological sequele to needling of lesions in the vertebrae [27].

Chapter 4

Cytology of Normal Constituents in Bone Aspirates and of Reactive Changes

Normal Cells in Bone Aspirates

The normal cells which may be present in bone aspirates are osteoblasts, osteoclasts, chondrocytes, bone marrow cells and mesothelial cells.

Osteoblasts

Osteoblasts are most often seen as single cells but small clusters or rows are also encountered. Osteoblasts are uniform cells, rounded or triangular, with abundant cytoplasm which typically contains an evident clear area or 'Hof' adjacent to the nucleus. Nuclei are rounded with a central nucleolus and are characteristically eccentrically situated close to the cytoplasmic membrane, almost protruding through it (fig. 3).

Osteoclasts

Osteoclasts always appear as single large cells with abundant cytoplasm and multiple uniform rounded nuclei, often arranged close together. A fine red cytoplasmic granulation is seen in air-dried smears stained with May-Grünwald Giemsa (MGG) or DiffQuick (fig. 4).

Chondrocytes

Normal chondrocytes are sometimes seen in bone aspirates, especially from lesions near joints and costochondral junctions. They are never seen as single cells but are present in lacunae in small, cartilaginous fragments. These fragments are composed of a hyaline-like matrix, red-blue to violet in MGG or DiffQuick smears and pink with hematoxylin and eosin staining. The matrix appears fibrillary and greyish-red

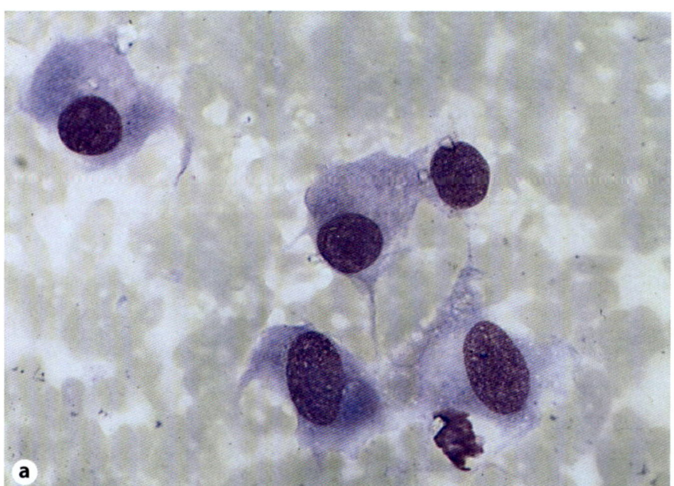

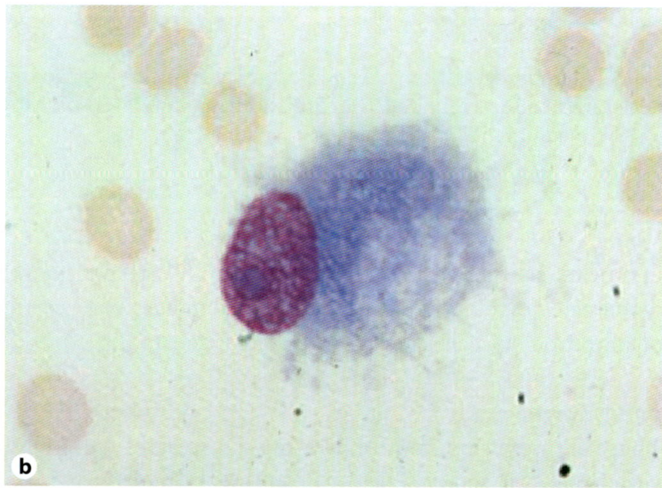

Fig. 3. Osteoblasts. The typical osteoblast is plasma cell-like, triangular or rounded, with rather abundant cytoplasm and an eccentric nucleus. A perinuclear clear 'Hof' is obvious in most cells. **a** MGG, medium magnification. **b** MGG, high magnification.

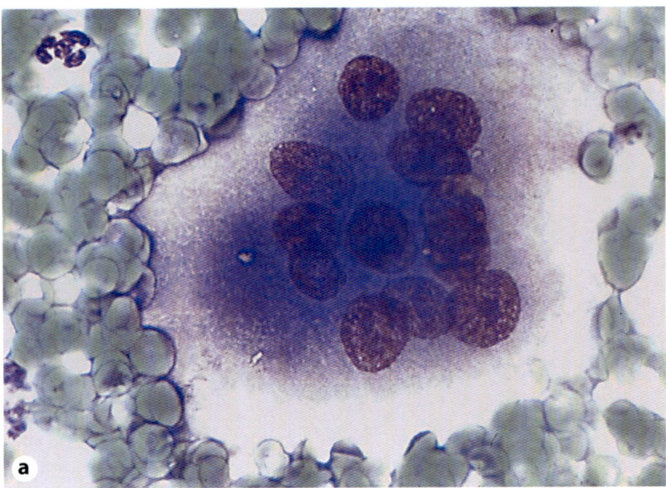
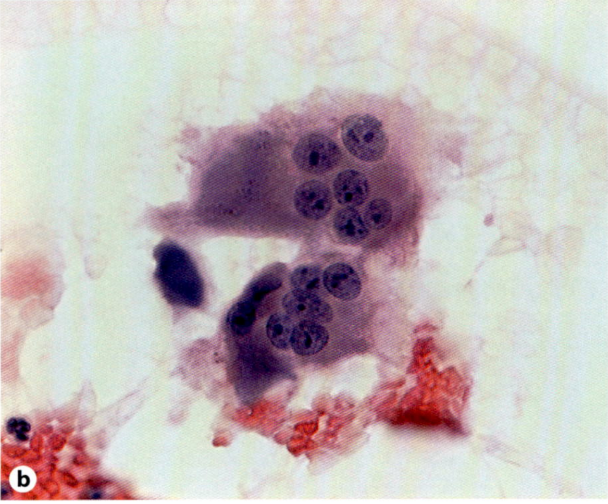

Fig. 4. Osteoclasts. Osteoclasts are large cells with abundant cytoplasm with a fine red granulation in MGG-stained smears. Osteoclasts possess at least 12–15 uniform rounded nuclei. **a** HE, high magnification. **b** MGG, high magnification.

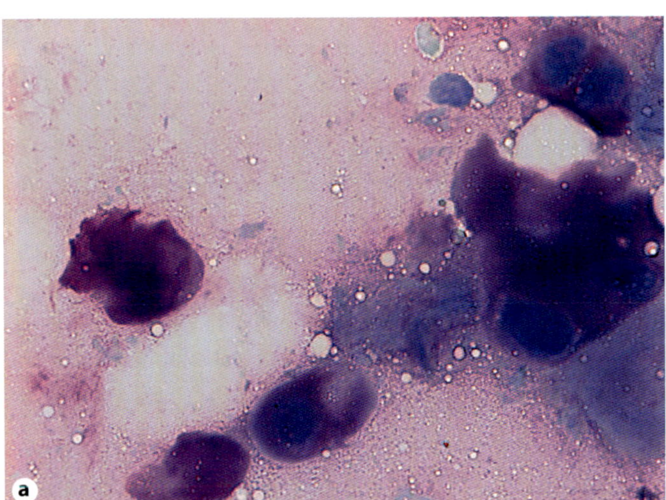
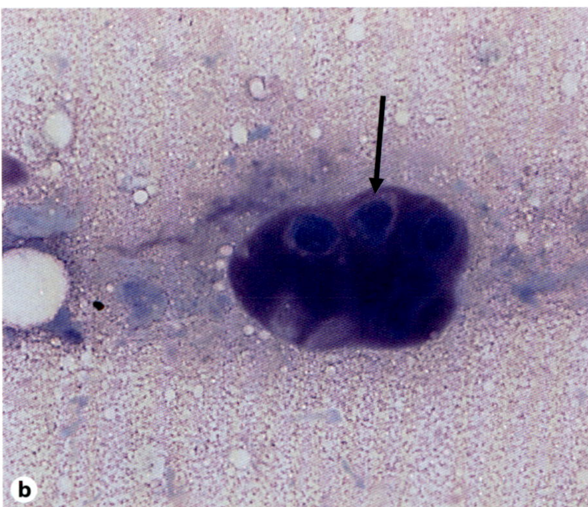

Fig. 5. Chondrocytes. Normal chondrocytes are typically seen in small cartilaginous fragments, often located within lacunae (arrow in **b**). The nuclei are small and rounded. The cartilaginous matrix is red-blue to violet in MGG-stained smears and red or pink in HE and Pap, respectively. **a** MGG, medium magnification. **b** MGG, medium magnification.

in smears stained with Pap. The chondrocytes have poorly demarcated cytoplasm and small rounded nuclei. The texture of chondrocytes is best seen in wet-fixed smears (fig. 5).

Bone Marrow Cells

These are a not uncommon finding in aspirates from ribs, vertebrae and sacrum. Most commonly there is a mixture of erythropoietic and myelopoietic cells and megakaryocytes. It is important not to misinterpret scattered megakaryocytes as malignant cells. The bone marrow cells are best identified in smears stained with MGG or DiffQuick (fig. 6).

Mesothelial Cells

Sheets of mesothelial cells are occasionally found in the smears when vertebral lesions are needled and the needle misses the target or penetrates through the vertebra. It is important not to misdiagnose reactive mesothelial cells as

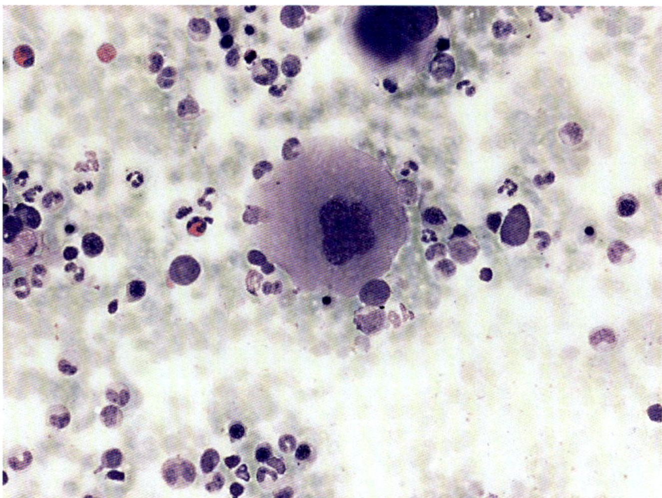

Fig. 6. Bone marrow cells. Most commonly, bone marrow in skeletal aspirates includes all 3 lineages (erythropoietic and myelopoietic cells and megakaryocytes). It is important not to misinterpret megakaryocytes as tumour cells when they appear as single cells on a haemorrhagic background. The bone marrow cells are best identified in MGG or DiffQuick-stained smears. MGG, medium magnification.

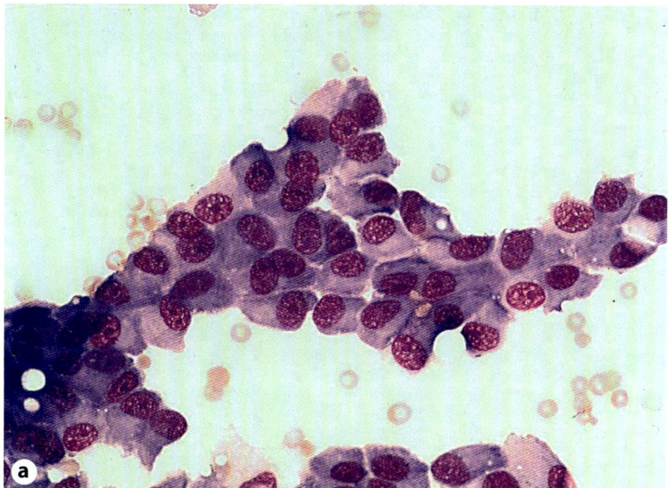

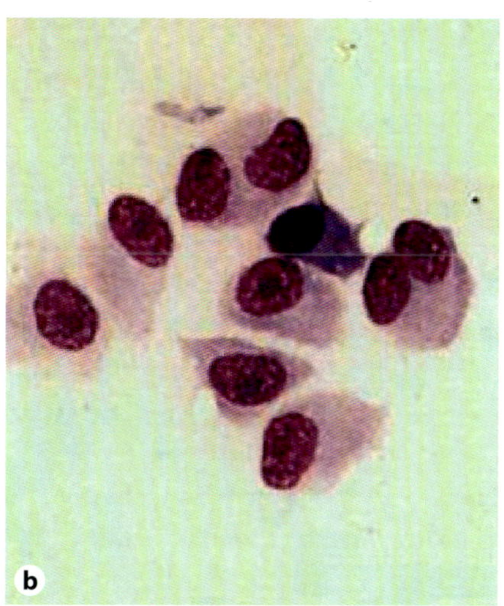

Fig. 7. Mesothelial cells. A clean background is the best criterion for mesothelial cells in aspirates from vertebral lesions. Only scattered erythrocytes are sometimes visible. All bone aspirates are generally haemorrhagic. **a** MGG, medium magnification. **b** MGG, high magnification.

adenocarcinoma cells. Bone aspirates, including those from the vertebrae are, as a rule, haemorrhagic but the smears usually have a clean, non-haemorrhagic background when only mesothelial cells are aspirated (fig. 7).

Reactive Changes

Reactive changes are only seen in osteoblasts and are found in smears from fracture callus and from proliferative periosteitis. The reactive osteoblasts resemble their normal counterparts and have eccentric nuclei and a cytoplasmic Hof but their size is variable and they show anisokaryosis and sometimes have prominent nucleoli (fig. 8).

Pseudomalignant Myositis Ossificans

This is a worrisome lesion exhibiting reactive osteoblasts as well as reactive myofibroblasts.

Pseudomalignant myositis ossificans (PMO) is a reactive, often self-healing lesion, characterized by heterotopic ossification.

It occurs predominantly in adolescents and young adults, typically after trauma but there is no history of injury in a number of cases. PMO is usually found deep in the extremities within striated muscle, sometimes close to the periostal surface. PMO might be clinically and radiologically interpreted as a lesion of the bone surface. Radiologically, mature lesions have a very characteristic zonal ossification pattern with a shell of calcifications at the periphery of a well-demarcated mass. The central part is histologically made up of fibrovascular tissue exhibiting reactive myofibroblasts, ganglion-cell-like large cells with prominent nucleoli, reactive osteoblasts and multinucleated osteoclast-like cells. Evidence of old haemorrhage may be seen. The cellular composition resembles a florid nodular fasciitis or proliferative fasciitis.

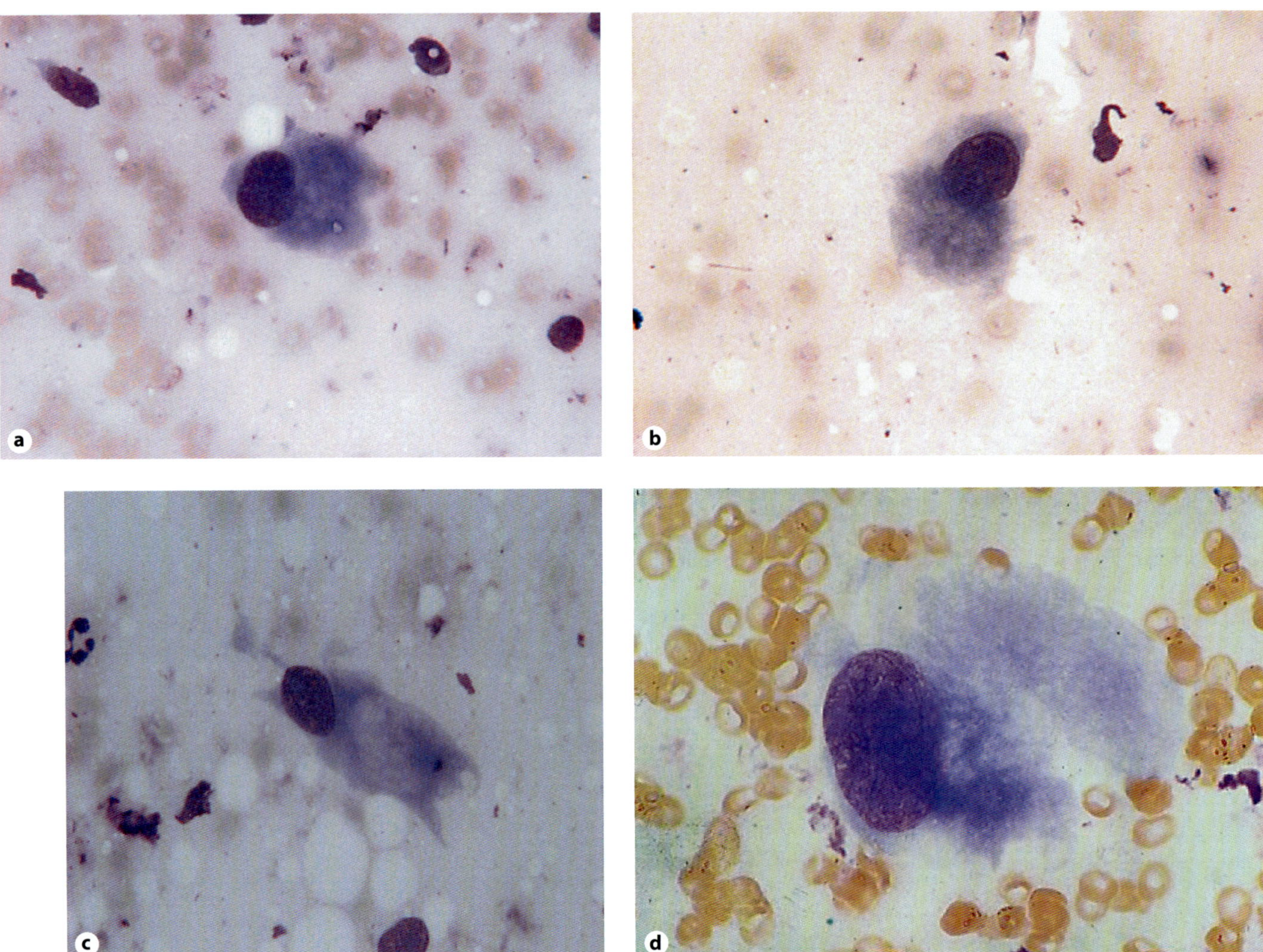

Fig. 8. Reactive osteoblasts. Reactive osteoblasts resemble normal osteoblasts; the nuclei are eccentric and a cytoplasmic 'Hof' is visible. Their size and shape are variable, anisokaryosis may be marked and nucleoli prominent. **a–d** Four reactive osteoblasts. MGG, high magnification.

The cytological features of PMO are (fig. 9):

- Osteoblast-like cells
- Proliferating myofibroblasts
- Osteoclast-like multinucleated giant cells
- Small calcifications (rare)

The differential diagnosis is osteosarcoma. The diagnosis of PMO should be based on the cytological pattern in combination with clinical and radiographic data. The zonal ossification pattern is an important diagnostic sign. Osteoid is not found and although the proliferating and reactive myofibroblasts and osteoblasts may present with marked anisokaryosis and prominent nucleoli, clearly malignant multinucleated giant cells are not found and the cellular pattern is principally similar to that seen in the early phase of nodular or proliferative faciitis, except that there is no myxoid background matrix. The cytological features of PMO have been presented in 2 small series [28, 29] In our series of 5 cases, the lesions diminished considerably in size within some weeks [28].

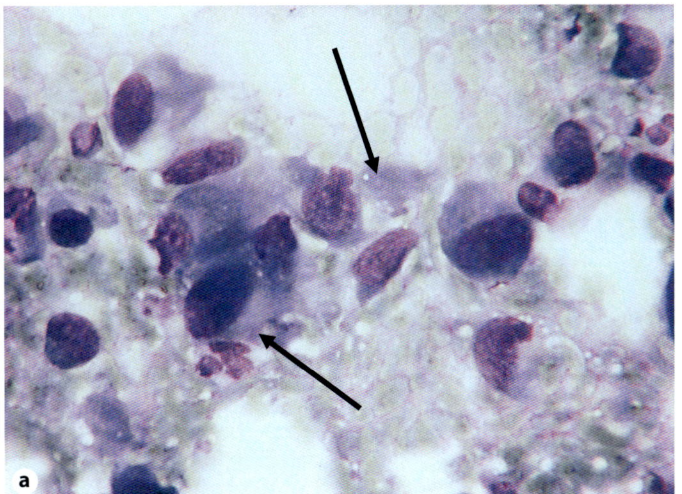

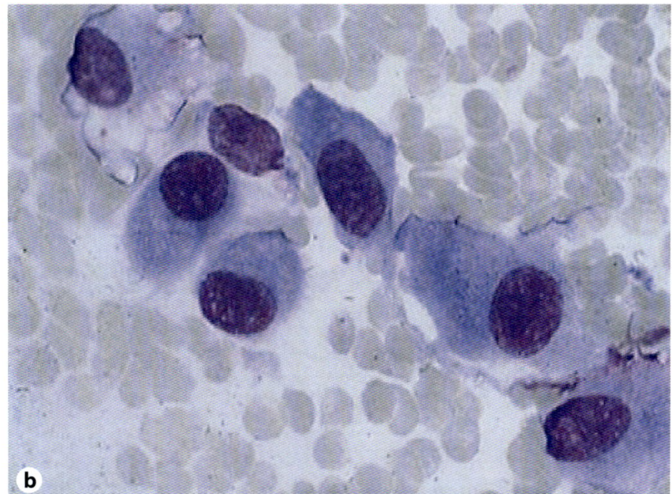

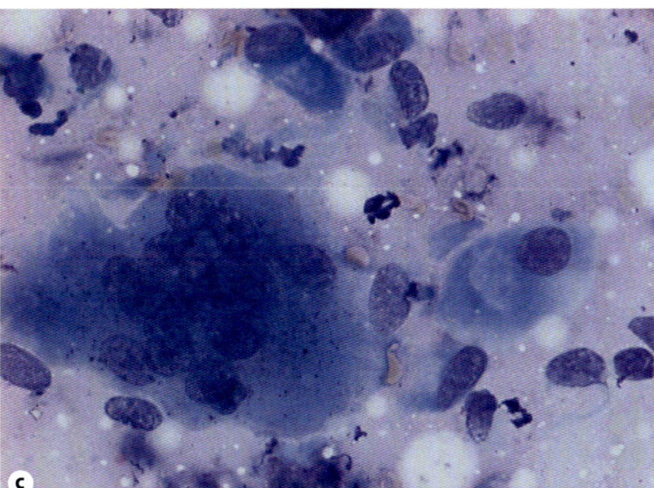

Fig. 9. Pseudomalignant myositis ossificans. **a** A mixture of reactive osteoblasts (arrow) and myofibroblasts. MGG, medium magnification. **b** Reactive osteoblasts. MGG, high magnification. **c** A multinucleated osteoclast-like giant cell and reactive osteoblasts. MGG, High magnification.

Chapter 5

Cytological Features of Bone Tumours in FNA Smears I: Osteogenic Tumours

Osteid Osteoma and Osteoblastoma

Osteid osteoma and osteoblastoma are benign osteoblastic tumours with overlapping radiographic and histological features. Osteid osteoma has distinctive clinical features and is almost never referred for fine needle aspiration cytology (FNAC). Due to the reactive, sclerotic bone surrounding the osteoma nidus this lesion is anyhow not suitable for FNAC.

Osteoblastoma is a rare benign tumour (<1% of bone tumours). Most patients are between 10 and 30 years of age and predilection sites are the spine and sacrum (up to 50% of cases). Of other sites, the proximal and distal femur and proximal tibia are the most frequent. The vast majority of osteoblastomas are intra-osseous tumours.

Radiology
The radiological signs are non-specific (fig. 10). The tumours are osteolytic, osteosclerotic or mixed. The bone may be expanded by the lesion with thinning of the cortex and a soft tissue component may also be present. In most cases the lesion is well circumscribed, and partially calcified and may look like a large osteoid osteoma. Osteoblastoma should be suspected in cases of this type. The lesions usually originate in the cortical or medullary bone, and only rarely in the subperiosteal region.

In the aggressive variant of osteoblastoma the radiological pattern is that of a malignant tumour (moth-eaten and permeative).

Histopathology
Osteoblastomas are composed of haphazardly arranged bone trabelulae or spiculae. The trabeculae are lined by osteoblasts, which may show anisokaryosis and mitoses, but no atypia. The tumours are vascular, and osteoclast-like multinucleated giant cells and small islands of osteoid are present between the bone trabeculae (fig. 11).

Aggressive osteoblastoma, a rare variant of osteoblastoma, is considered as a borderline tumour between conventional osteoblastoma and osteosarcoma. Aggressive osteoblastomas do not metastasize but recurrences are not unusual. The typical hallmark of aggressive osteoblastoma is the so-called epithelioid osteoblasts. These cells are larger than ordinary osteoblasts, have an abundant cytoplasm and large rounded or ovoid nuclei with prominent nucleoli. A clear cytoplasmic 'Hof' is often present. The epithelioid osteoblasts often form cohesive clusters [2]. Epithelioid osteoblastoma is an alternative term proposed for aggressive osteoblastoma [30].

Cytological Features of Osteoblastoma
These are shown in figure 12. Features include: osteoblast-like cells, mononucleted and binucleated, which are alone or in small clusters; large osteoclast-like multinucleated giant cells, and small clusters or groups of spindle cells.

Differential Diagnosis
The differential diagnosis is osteosarcoma.

Comments
Only very few cases of FNAC of osteoblastoma have been recorded [31, 32]. Our experience is limited to single cases. We consider, however, that conventional osteoblastoma is possible to diagnose cytologically as a benign primary bone tumour because neither the osteoblasts nor the multinucleated osteoclast-like giant cells exhibit malignant features. Cytological criteria have not been defined for the diagnosis of aggressive (epithelioid) osteoblastoma in FNA smears.

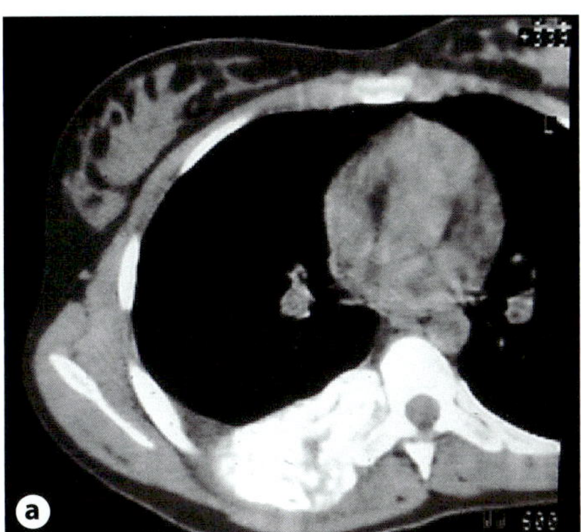

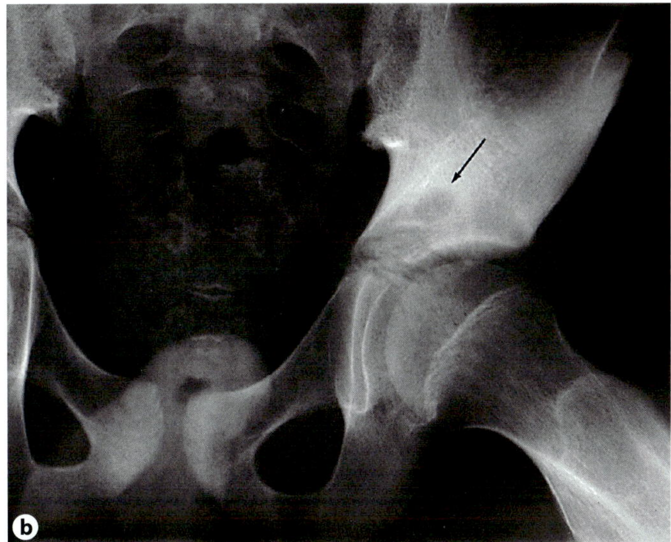

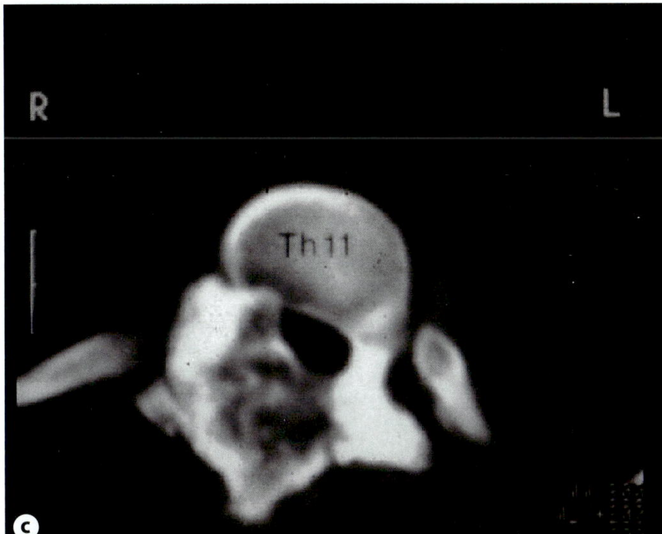

Fig. 10. Osteoblastoma. Radiologic features. **a** CT of the thorax. There is an extensive osteoblastoma of the medial aspect of a rib. The lesion is sclerotic and expansile. **b** AP radiograph of the pelvis and left hip joint. There is a lytic lesion in the acetabulum surrounded by sclerosis (arrow). The lesion is non-specific, but the findings are compatible with an osteoblastoma. **c** CT of the eleventh thoracic vertebra. A large lesion of the right pedicle and lamina of the vertebra is evident. There is central lysis surrounded by sclerosis.

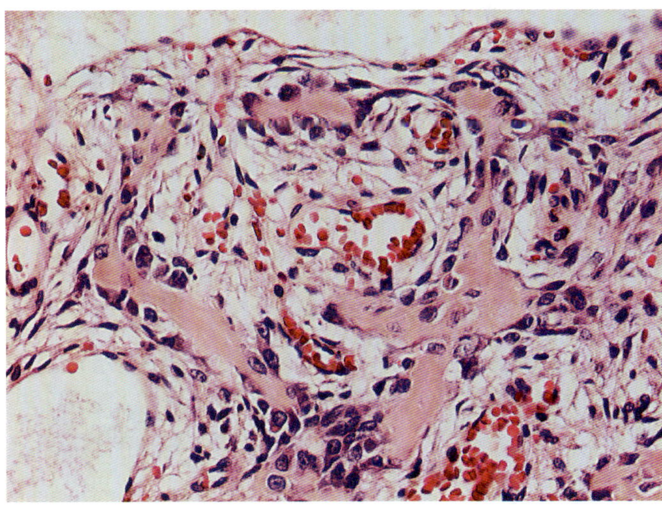

Fig. 11. Osteoblastoma. Histology. Bone trabeculae bordered by moderately pleomorphic osteoblasts and scattered osteoclasts in a vascular stroma. HE, medium magnification.

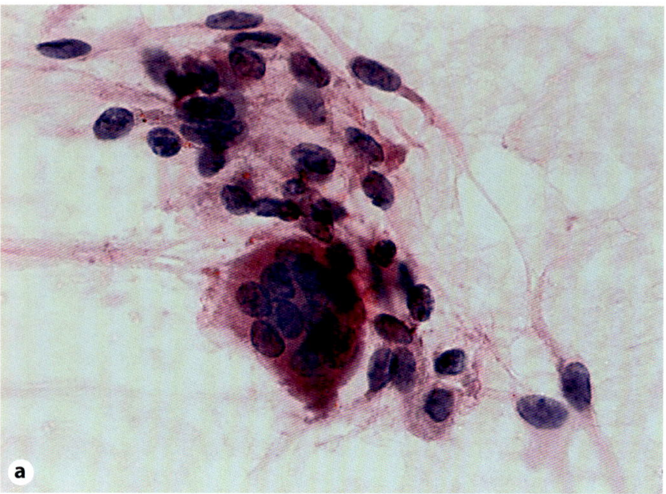

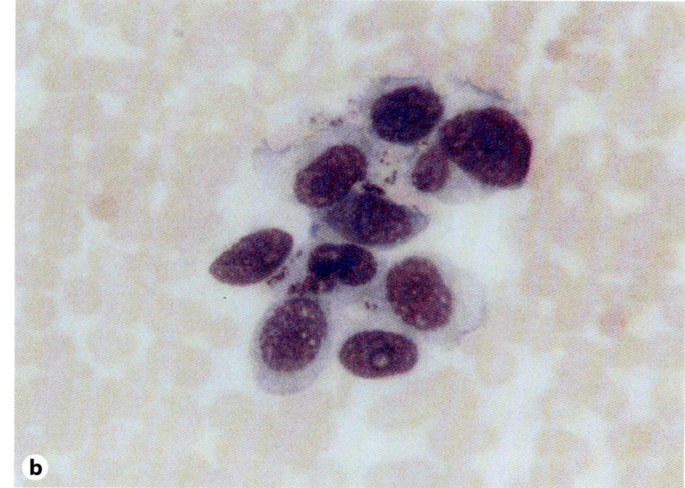

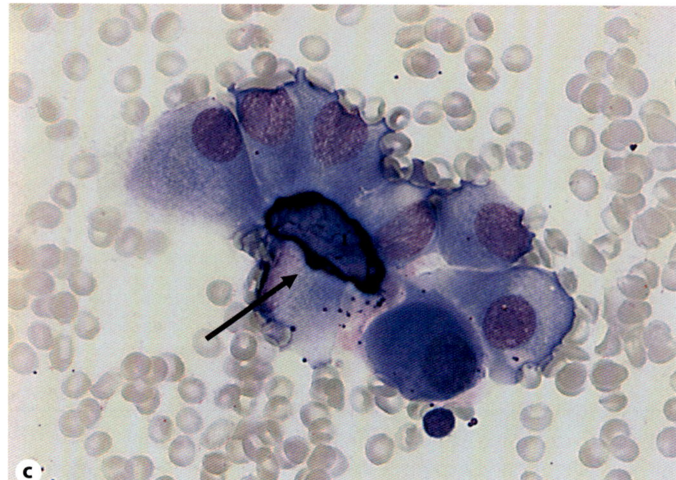

Fig. 12. Osteoblastoma. **a** A cluster of osteoblasts and spindle cells. An osteoclast-like giant cell is in the lower left corner. HE, medium magnification. **b**, **c** Small groups of osteoblasts. A small calcification is seen in **c** (arrow). MGG, high magnification.

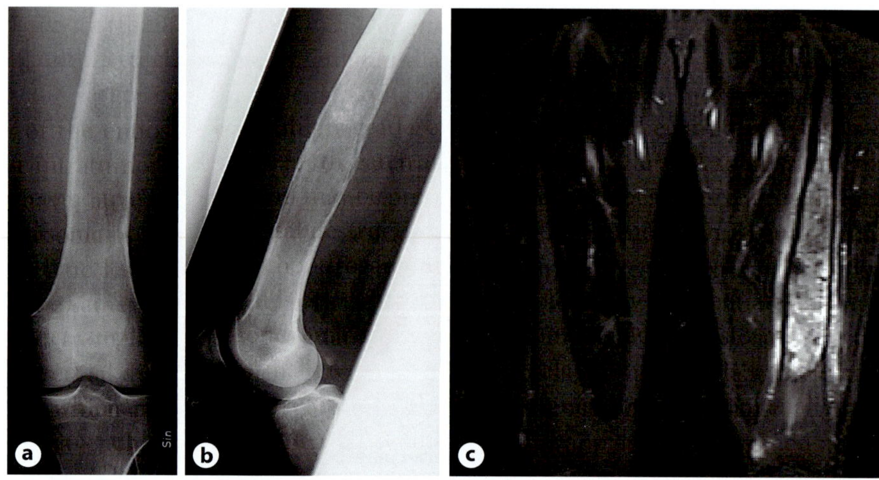

Fig. 13. Osteosarcoma. Radiologic features. **a**, **b** AP and lateral radiograph of the left femur. There is a lytic, expansile lesion of the distal diaphysis of the femur, with thinning of the cortex and laminated periosteal reaction. The character of the lesion is that of a malignant tumour, but the location is atypical for osteosarcoma. **c**. Coronar MRI of the femur, STIR sequence. The lesion in the bone marrow has a high signal. The soft tissues medial and lateral to the femur also have a high signal, although only seen as a thin rim in this section.

A primary bone tumour featuring clearly atypical, large osteoblasts with prominent nucleoli should be diagnosed as inconclusive in regard to benign osteoblastoma or osteosarcoma, irrespective of the radiological features.

Osteosarcoma

Osteosarcoma is a primary bone tumour composed of cells, which at least focally produce tumoral bone (osteoid). Excluding plasmocytoma/myeloma, osteosarcoma is the most frequent primary malignant bone tumour and is considered twice as common as chondrosarcoma. The majority of patients are in their second decade. A second peak (10%) occurs in patients around 60 years of age. Osteosarcoma is rare in young children and even rarer in infants. The most common symptoms are pain and a palpable bone mass, often with a soft tissue extension. Any bone in the body may harbour an osteosarcoma, with the most typical sites being around the knee followed by the humerus and pelvic bones. Approximately 7–10% arise in the craniofascial bones (maxilla and mandible). Osteosarcoma is rare in the spine and in the small bones of hands and feet.

Osteosarcomas show a wide variation both in regard to location in the bone and to their morphological appearance. The conventional intramedullary subtype is the most common. Less common variants are periosteal osteosarcoma, parosteal or juxtacortical osteosarcoma, central low-grade osteosarcoma, high-grade surface osteosarcoma and small-cell osteosarcoma.

Radiology

The radiological characteristics of osteosarcomas are variable (fig. 13). The most common appearance is an ill-defined lytic intramedullary lesion with destruction of the overlying cortical bone. A periosteal reaction with Codman's triangle and a 'sunburst' appearance is commonly seen adjacent to the tumour. Intramedullary lesions with minor cortical destruction may feature a periosteal reaction of the 'onion peel' appearance.

Osteosarcomas may also be sclerotic with matrix calcification. A mixed pattern with both lytic and sclerotic areas is also common. In all these patterns, a soft tissue component is almost mandatory. The soft tissue extension is best shown with CT or MRI. In the early stage, the radiographic appearance may be subtle and easy to overlook. A subtle periosteal reaction and Codman's triangle are important signs that should lead to further investigations. Plain radiography is important as a screening method but the extent and grading is made on MRI. The bone marrow extension is best shown on MRI, as are the so-called skip lesions (local metastases in the same bone, at times occurring quite distant to the primary lesion). It is thus important to examine the whole bone that contains the tumour. Distant metastases are best discovered by bone scintigraphy or total body MRI. Lung metastases are best visualized with CT.

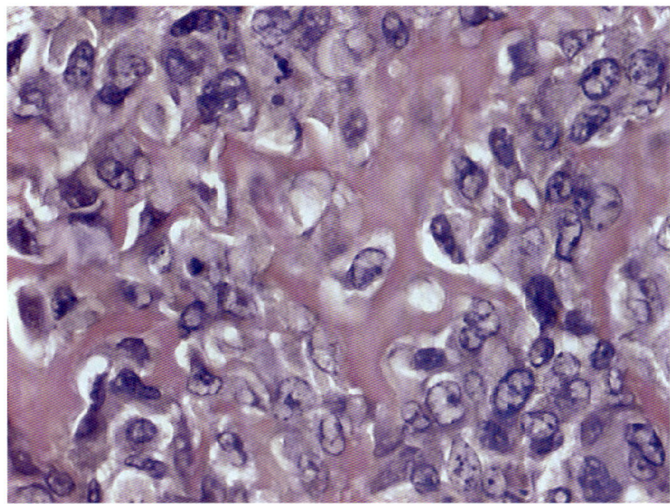

Fig. 14. Osteoblastic osteosarcoma. Histology. Large, atypical tumour cells with irregular nuclei and moderate amount of cytoplasm. Intercellular strands of osteoid matrix. HE, medium magnification.

The characteristics of the tumour matrix can be evaluated with contrast medium enhanced MRI. Normally there is enhancement of the tumour. When part(s) of the tumour does not enhance, this suggests necrosis (and/or intratumoral haemorrhage). It is a valuable piece of information in cases where image-guided FNA is planned.

Parosteal osteosarcoma is sclerotic, extending from the cortex like a root from which the tumour grows like a mushroom along and/or around the bone. CT often demonstrates a cleavage plane between the sclerotic tumour and the cortical bone.

Histopathology

The histological classification in osteoblastic, chondroblastic and fibroblastic variants was proposed by Dahlin more than 30 years ago and is still widely used. In conventional intramedullary osteosarcoma, all forms show marked cellular and nuclear pleomorphism, atypical mitoses and foci of more or less mineralized osteoid (fig. 14). Foci of malignant cartilage are present in chondroblastic osteosarcoma, while the fibroblastic variant is made up of atypical spindle cells mimicking fibrosarcoma. The tumour cells may look like

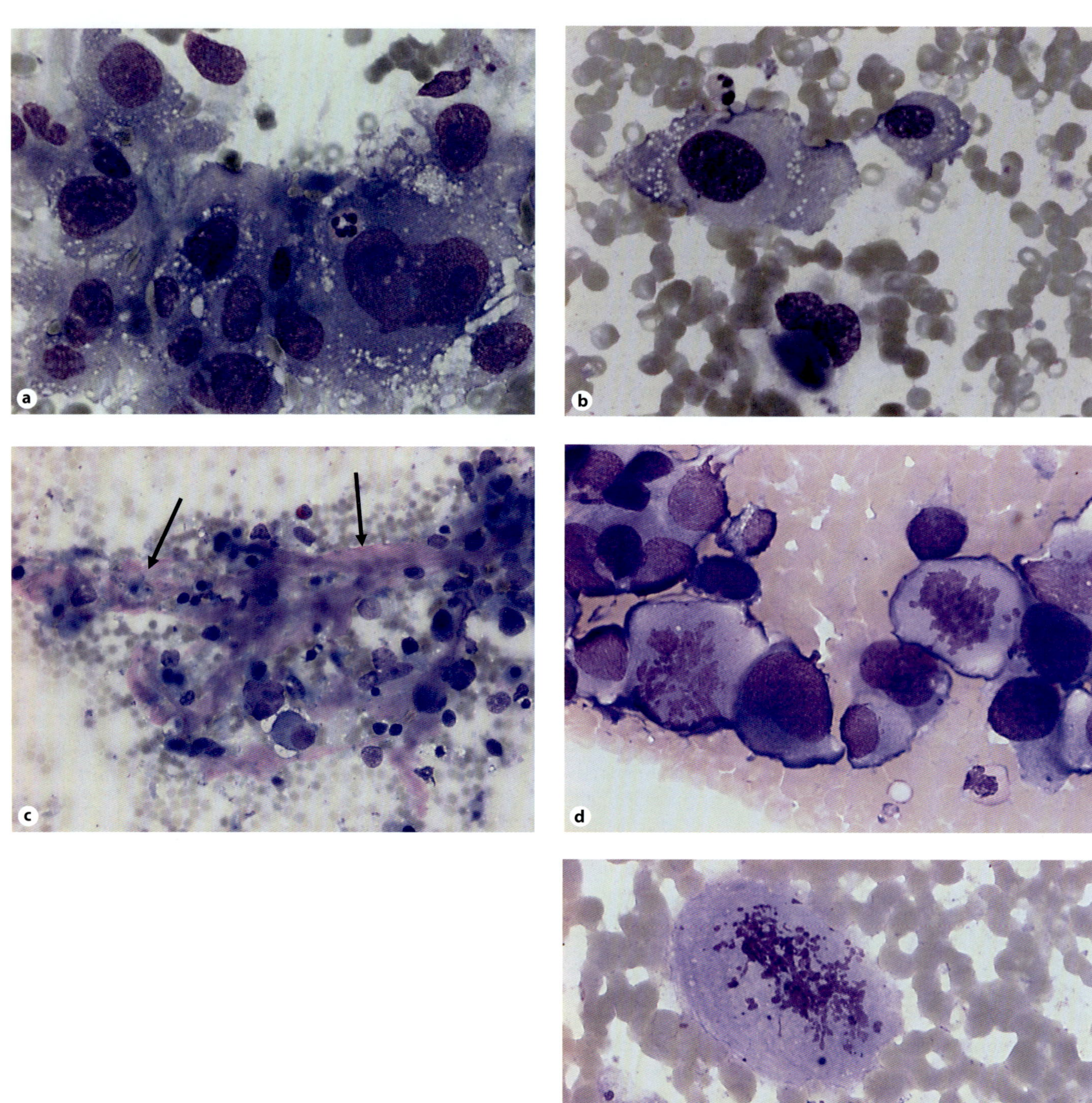

Fig. 15. Osteoblastic osteosarcoma. **a**, **b** Large tumour cells with rounded nuclei and a variable amount of cytoplasm. MGG, high magnification. **c** Thin strands of osteoid matrix between the tumour cells. MGG, medium magnification. **d**, **e** Atypical mitoses are not seldom observed. MGG, high magnification.

highly atypical osteoblasts or have an epithelioid appearance. Tumour giant cells are not uncommon.

Telangiectatic osteosarcoma occurs in the same sites as conventional osteosarcoma. It often appears as a blood-filled cavity and may simulate an aneurysmal bone cyst. Malignant cells are present in the blood and line the walls of the cavities. There are often numerous osteoclast-like giant cells and foci of siderophages. A high mitotic rate with atypical mitoses is a common finding. Numerous multinucleated benign giant cells are also present in the so-called giant-cell-rich osteosarcoma. A subset of conventional osteosarcoma may resemble osteoblastoma within large areas. This is a diagnostically worrisome variant in which the growth pattern (permeation of surrounding tissues with presence of entrapped normal bone) is an important diagnostic sign [33].

Parosteal osteosarcomas are relatively rare (approx. 5% of all osteosarcomas). They are metaphyseal tumours, predominantly localized to the femur. They are most commonly hypocellular, made up of slightly atypical spindle cells exhibiting a low mitotic rate. Low-grade malignant cartilaginous areas are present in up to 50% of cases. The small-cell osteosarcoma is also relatively rare (approx. 4% of all osteosarcomas). The predilection sites are the metaphyses of the long bones. Histologically, sheets of small rounded or spindly cells producing osteoid matrix are the main feature. The tumour cell nuclei are rounded or ovoid with finely granular chromatin resembling the cells of conventional Ewing's sarcoma. Foci of neoplastic cartilage may be present. The periosteal osteosarcoma is another rare variant (approx. 1–2% of all osteosarcomas). It arises most commonly in the diaphyses of the tibia or femur. The tumour shows a predominance of chondroid areas, osteoid is usually scanty and calcifications are present. The central low-grade osteosarcoma is as rare as the periosteal type. It is most often situated in the metaphyses of the femur and tibia. The tumours are often collagen-rich, with sheets of slightly atypical spindle cells. The mitotic rate is low. The high-grade surface osteosarcoma is extremely rare (only 0.6% of all osteosarcomas). It arises from the deep layers of the periosteum, most commonly in the femur or humerus.

Conventional osteosarcoma, including the giant-cell-rich and teleangiectatic varietes are the most commonly aspirated osteosarcomas. The relatively numerous series of cases reporting the cytological features have been mainly of conventional osteosarcomas [31, 34–38]. In our reported series of 59 osteosarcomas diagnosed by FNAC, the final diagnosis was teleangiectatic osteosarcoma in 4 patients, 2 had high-grade surface osteosarcoma, 1 had a giant-cell-rich osteosarcoma and 2 presented with parosteal osteosarcoma [37]. We also have a case of small-cell osteosarcoma in our files. To our knowledge, there are no reports of the cytological features of periosteal and central low-grade osteosarcoma.

Cytological Features

Osteoblastic Subtype. See figure 15. This subtype shows variable cellularity, with a mixture of single cells and clusters in moderately cellular smears. Tumour cells are moderately to highly pleomorphic, rounded, ovoid, polygonal and often large. The pleomorphic tumour cells may be osteoblast-like with eccentric nuclei and a faint cytoplasmic Hof. Clustered tumour cells may be epithelioid with distinct sharp cytoplasmic borders and rounded nuclei with prominent nucleoli. There are multinucleated tumour giant cells. Strands of osteoid matrix [staining red or purple in May-Grünwald Giemsa (MGG), pale pink in hematoxylin and eosin (HE)] exist between tumour cells in clusters. There is frequent mitoses, which are often atypical. Benign osteoclast-like giant cells are numerous in giant-cell-rich osteosarcoma. Occasional necrosis and calcifications are seen.

Chondroblastic Subtype. See figure 16. This subtype has a myxoid background matrix (staining red or red-violett in MGG). There is an admixture of dispersed atypical mono- or binucleated chondroblast-like tumour cells, in addition to a similar cell population as seen in osteoblastic osteosarcoma. Occasionally fragments of hyaline cartilage with atypical cells in lacunae are seen.

Fibroblastic Subtype. See figure 17. The fibroblastic subtype shows predominance of atypical spindle-shaped cells with cytoplasmic processes and coarse nuclear chromatin. Strands of osteoid less common.

Parosteal Osteosarcoma. There are fragments of hyaline cartilage with slightly atypical cells. Strands of slightly atypical spindly cells.

Small-Cell Osteosarcoma. See figure 18. This osteosarcoma shows a mixture of clustered and dispersed small to medium-sized rounded or spindly cells. The rounded tumour cell nuclei have finely granular chromatin and inconspicuous nucleoli. There are fragments of hyaline cartilage. The presence of osteoid matrix is less common.

Differential Diagnosis

There are a number of possible differential diagnoses: reactive osteoblastic proliferations, as in fracture callus and pseudomalignant myositis ossificans; osteoblastoma; giant-cell tumour (giant-cell-rich osteosarcoma, teleangiectatic osteosarcoma); aneurysmal bone cyst (telangiectatic

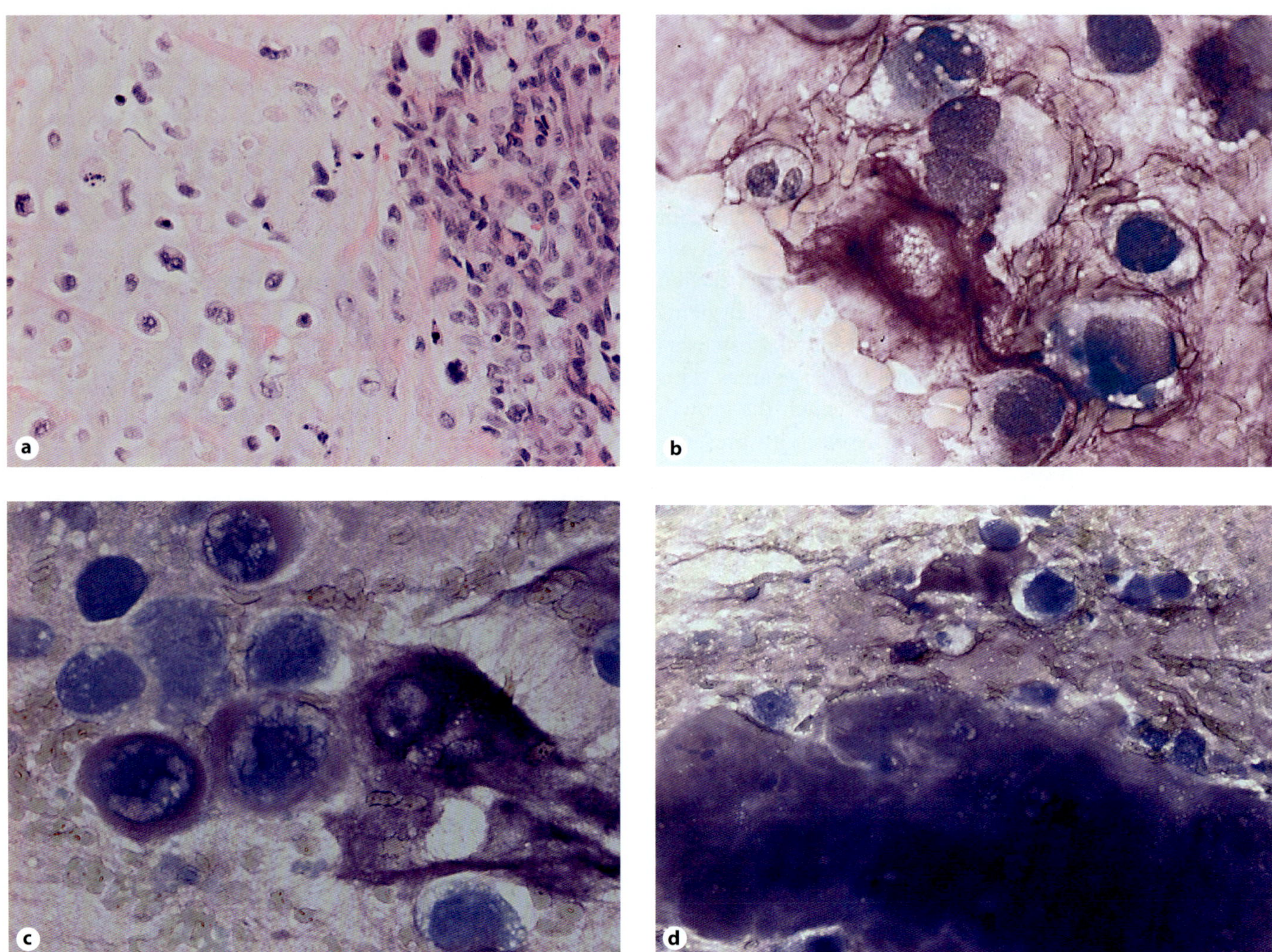

Fig. 16. Chondroblastic osteosarcoma. **a** Atypical cartilaginous tissue with tumour cells in lacunae is present to the left in this histologic section. HE, low magnification. **b–d** Large, atypical tumour cells embedded in a chondroid matrix that stains variably red, violet and blue. This matrix is more abundant than osteoid matrix in pure osteoblastic osteosarcoma. MGG, medium magnification.

osteosarcoma); high-grade malignant chondrosarcoma; pleomorphic sarcoma (malignant fibrous histiocytoma-type, pleomorphic leiomyosarcoma); conventional Ewing's sarcoma (small-cell osteosarcoma); mesenchymal chondrosarcoma (small-cell osteosarcoma); primary large-cell anaplastic lymphoma in bone; metastatic carcinoma; metastatic melanoma.

Comments

Although osteosarcoma is the primary bone sarcoma in which FNA cytology has been most thoroughly investigated, in a total of 223 cases, there are a number of important diagnostic pitfalls.

Reactive osteoblasts may be pleomorphic showing anisokaryosis and prominent nucleoli, but their chromatin pattern is regular and the cytoplasmic Hof clearly visible.

When the yield is poor and haemorrhagic, as may be the case in aspirates from telangiectatic osteosarcoma, osteoclast-like benign giant cells may predominate and scattered obviously malignant cells may be overlooked and there is a risk that the lesion could be misdiagnosed as an aneurysmal bone cyst.

In addition, the multinucleated benign giant cells present in giant-cell-rich osteosarcoma may be as numerous as in smears from giant-cell tumours. It is important to look for obvious malignant cells and atypical mitoses.

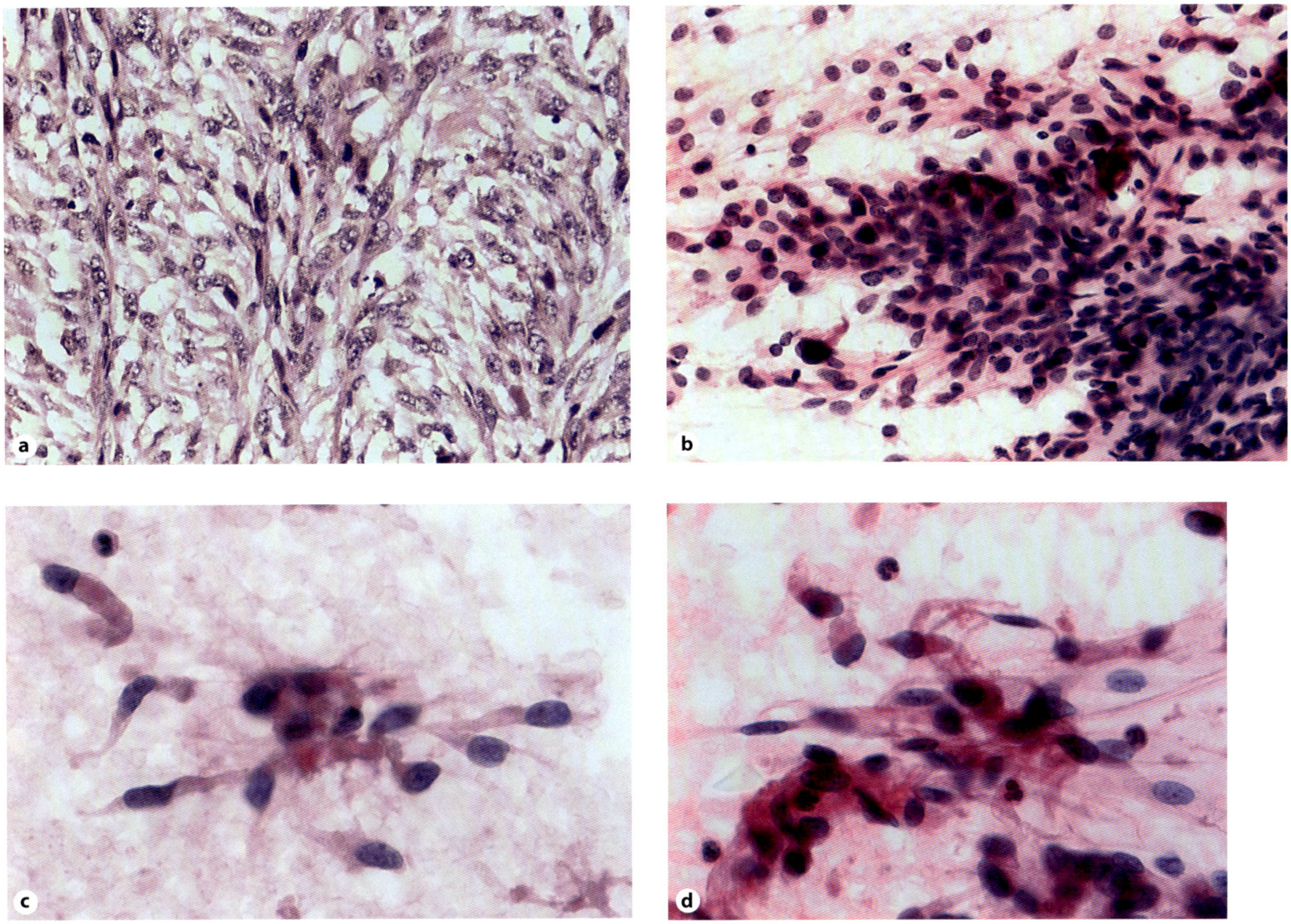

Fig. 17. Fibroblastic osteosarcoma. **a**. A section from a fibroblastic osteosarcoma with predominance of spindle-shaped tumour cells. HE, low magnification. **b–d**. The typical features of fibroblastic osteosarcoma in smears are groups or clusters of moderately atypical spindly cells with unipolar or bipolar cytoplasmic processes. **b** HE, low magnification. **c**, **d** HE, medium magnification.

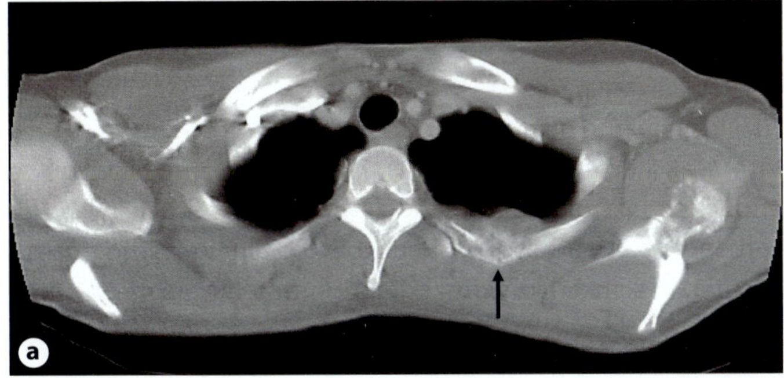

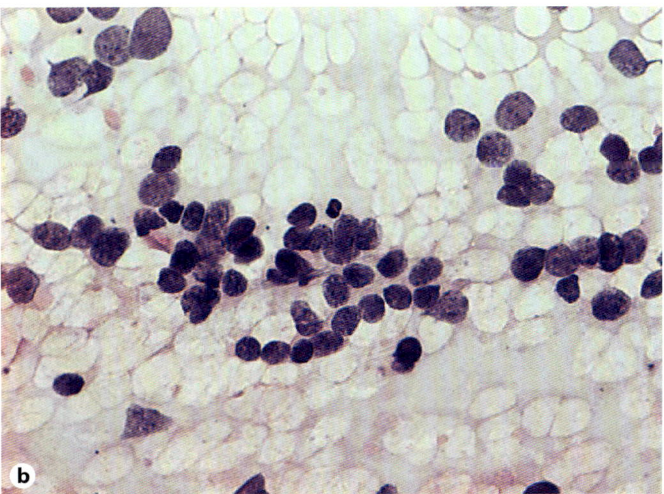

Fig. 18. Small-cell osteosarcoma. Radiological features. **a**. Transverse CT of the upper thorax. There is a lytic destruction in the left second rib, with pleural thickening overlying the bony destruction. **b** A cluster of partly cohesive small to medium sized tumour cells with moderately atypical rounded nuclei and scanty cytoplasm. When typical osteoid matrix is not found, a Ewing family tumour is a major differential diagnosis. HE, medium magnification.

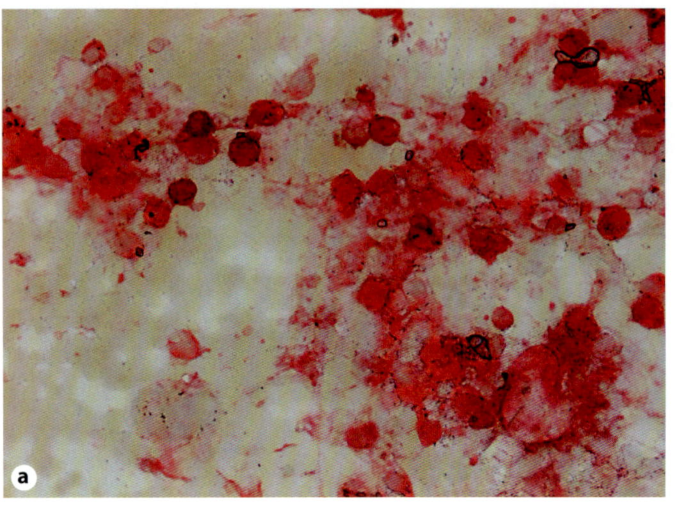

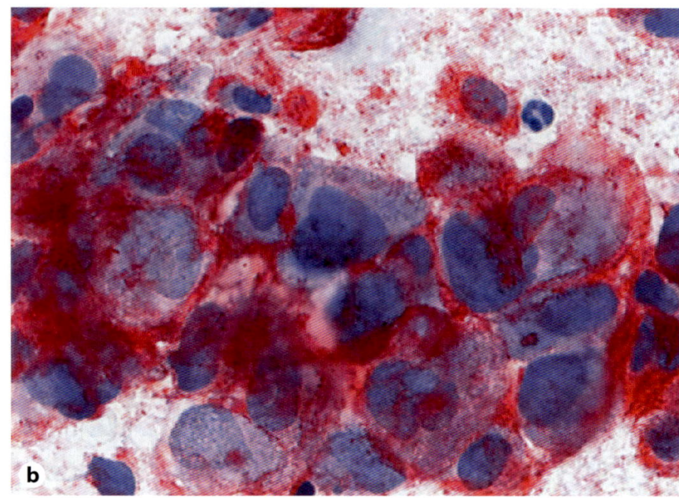

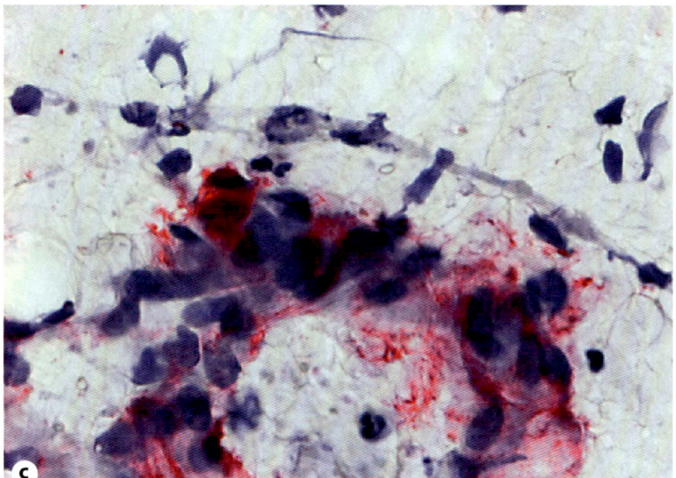

Fig. 19. ALP staining. The demonstration of cytoplasmic ALP is a major diagnostic adjunct. **a** Cytospin preparation. Low magnification. **b** Direct smear preparation. Medium magnification. **c**. Positive ALP-staining in a small-cell osteosarcoma. Cytospin preparation. Medium magnification.

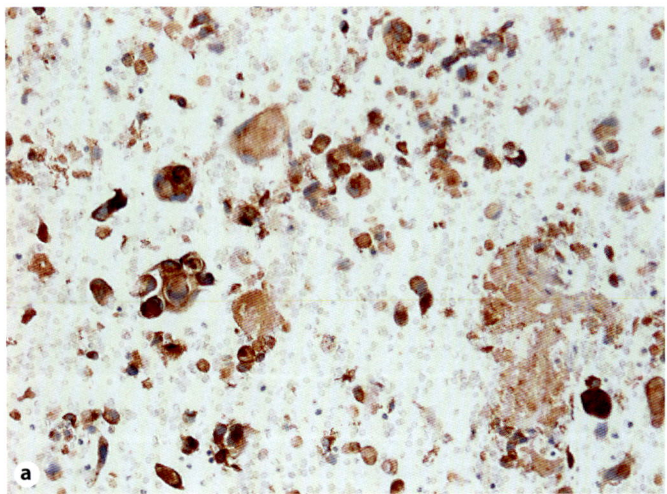

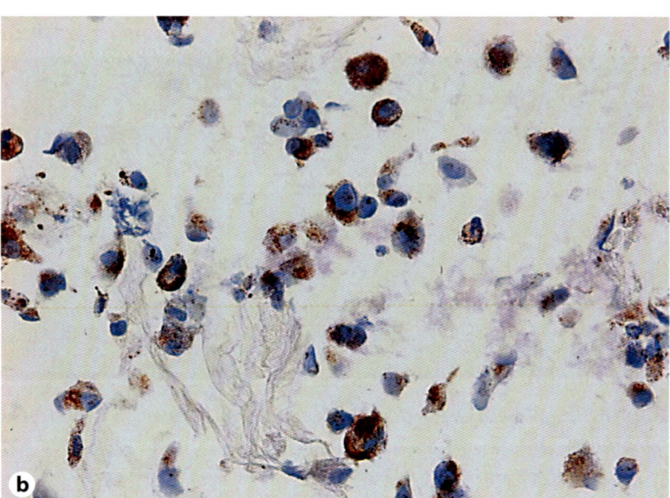

Fig. 20. Osteonectin. Immunoperoxidase, low magnification. Cell block preparation (**a**) and liquid-based (ThinPrep) preparation (**b**).

Osteoblastoma-like osteosarcoma is a diagnostic challenge in biopsy samples [33] and even more so in FNA material. When the radiological features in these cases are not unequivocally malignant, the cytological diagnosis is better reported as inconclusive than suspicious for osteosarcoma.

Another potential pitfall is that smears from chondroblastic osteosarcoma with excess of malignant cartilage might easily be misinterpreted as originating from a high-grade malignant chondrosarcoma.

When intercellular strands of osteoid are not present in the smears, the pleomorphic, markedly atypical cell population might be interpreted as representing one of the rare pleomorphic sarcomas (malignant fibrous histiocytoma type or pleomorphic leiomyosarcoma) arising de novo in bone. It is to be remembered that smears from pleomorphic leiomyosarcoma often contain osteoclast-like multinucleated cells.

The tumour cells of conventional osteosarcoma may exhibit epithelioid features such as distinct cell borders and rounded or ovoid nuclei with prominent nucleoli, and when they are clustered they can mimic cells from metastatic large-cell carcinoma.

Anaplastic large cell lymphoma can arise primarily in bone and may feature large cytoplasm-rich, rounded cells with eccentric nuclei and prominent nucleoli resembling highly atypical osteoblast-like tumour cells.

The clue to the cytological diagnosis of conventional osteosarcoma in routinely stained smears is the presence of intercellular osteoid and osteoblast-like tumour cells. Osteoid is best appreciated in MGG-stained smears.

It is at times necessary to supplement the routine stains with ancillary techniques to confirm or refute a diagnosis of conventional osteosarcoma. As stated in Chapter 3, strong intracytoplasmatic alkaline phosphatase staining (ALP) in intact tumour cells confirms their osteoblastic differentiation. ALP staining is of great help in the differential diagnosis between chondroblastic osteosarcoma and high-grade malignant (grade III) chondrosarcoma, as well as in the distinction from metastatic carcinoma or melanoma and from anaplastic large-cell lymphoma (fig. 19). Although not entirely specific for osteoblastic differentiation, a positive staining for osteonectin and osteocalcin strongly favours osteoblastic differentiation (fig. 20) [39, 40].

Differentiating osteoid from collagenous matrix can occasionally be difficult. Electron microscopic examination, however, is a well established method to define osteoid in fine needle aspirates [31].

DNA ploidy analysis is yet another valuable diagnostic complement. As stated earlier, conventional osteosarcomas usually are non-diploid while reactive osteoblasts are diploid. An unequivocal non-diploid histogram excludes a benign osteoblastic proliferation.

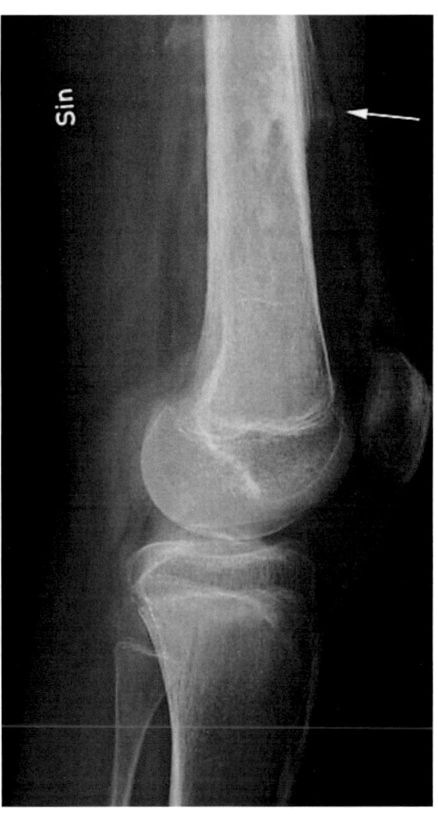

Fig. 21. Radiological features. Lateral view of the left femur showing no obvious bone destruction, but there is a periosteal reaction anteriorly. A Codman's triangle (arrow) indicates tumour growth outside the cortex with lifting of the periosteum. The nature of the lesion is non-specific although an osteosarcoma is the most likely.

Small-cell osteosarcoma may be difficult to distinguish from conventional Ewing's sarcoma and mesenchymal chondrosarcoma. In these 3 entities the tumour cells per se are very alike with scanty cytoplasm and bland nuclei with inconspicuous nucleoli. Osteoid matrix is less commonly found in small-cell osteosarcoma smears than fragments of hyaline matrix which makes the distinction from mesenchymal chondrosarcoma difficult.

Typical smears from conventional Ewing's sarcoma, however, do not contain matrix fragments and display a double cell population (large light and small dark cells). Immunocytochemistry is of limited value in the differential diagnosis since the CD99 antibody, considered as a hallmark antibody for the Ewing family of tumours, also marks the tumour cells in small-cell osteosarcoma and in mesenchymal chondrosarcoma.

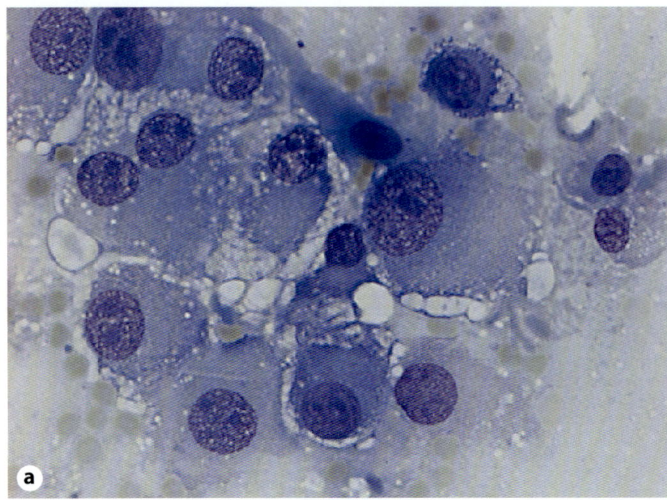

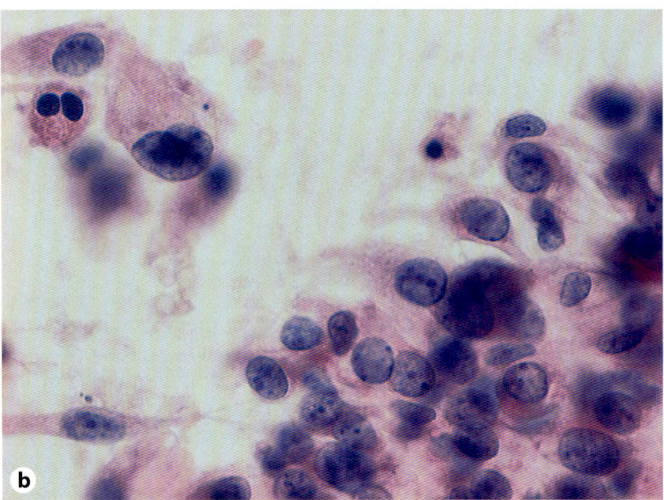

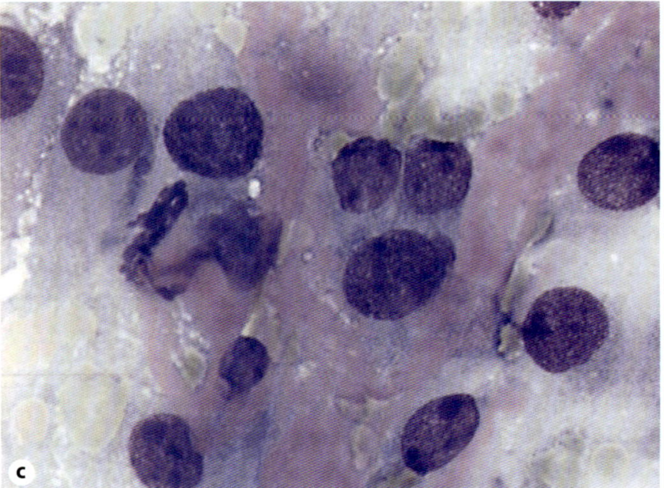

However, the translocation t(11;22), typical for the Ewing family of tumours, is not present in small-cell osteosarcoma [30]. FNAC of small-cell osteosarcoma has been presented in 1 case report [41].

Two important criteria for a diagnosis of small-cell osteosarcoma are positive ALP staining and immunoreactivity for osteonectin.

Case Report 1

The patients was a young male who reported pain in the distal part of the left thigh. On radiology (fig. 21), from a lateral view of the left femur there was no obvious bone destruction, but there was a periosteal reaction anteriorly. A Codman's triangle (arrow in the figure) indicated permeative tumour growth outside the cortex, with lifting of the periosteum. The nature of the lesion was non-specific, although an osteosarcoma was the first suggestion.

FNA was performed by the radiologist. Figure 22a (MGG, high magnification) and figure 22b (HE, high magnification) show cellular smears that were composed of large obviously malignant cells with abundant cytoplasm and eccentric nuclei with prominent nucleoli. Although there was no cytoplasmic Hof, the tumour cells looked like highly atypical osteoblasts. Figure 22c (MGG, high magnification) shows a cluster of loosely attached tumour cells with strands of a red/violet matrix, corresponding to osteoid (arrow), between the cells.

A preliminary diagnosis of osteoblastic osteosarcoma was rendered.

Figure 23a (HE, high magnification) shows part of a cell block preparation from the aspirate with well preserved tumour cells. Figure 23b (immunoperoxidase, high magnification) shows 1 large, osteoblast-like tumour cell positive for osteonectin.

The final cytological diagnosis was osteoblastic osteosarcoma.

Fig. 22. Cellular smears composed of large, obviously malignant, cells with abundant cytoplasm and eccentric nuclei with prominent nucleoli. Although there is no evident cytoplasmic Hof, the tumour cells look like highly atypical osteoblasts. **a** MGG, high magnification. **b** HE, high magnification. **c** A cluster of loosely cohesive tumour cells with intercellular strands of a red-violet matrix, corresponding to osteoid between the cells. MGG, high magnification.

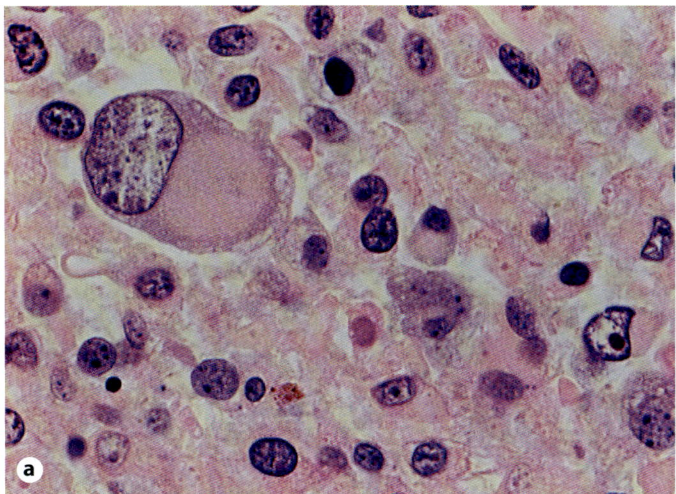

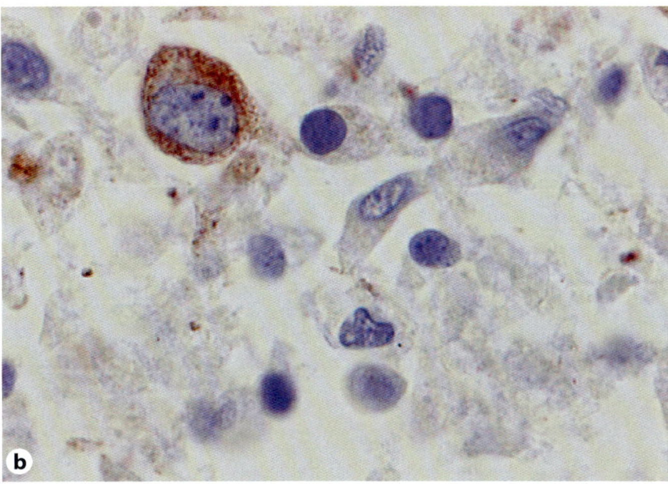

Fig. 23. a Part of a cell block preparation from the aspirate with well preserved tumour cells. HE, high magnification. **b** One large, osteoblast-like tumour cell positive for osteonectin. Immunoperoxidase, high magnification.

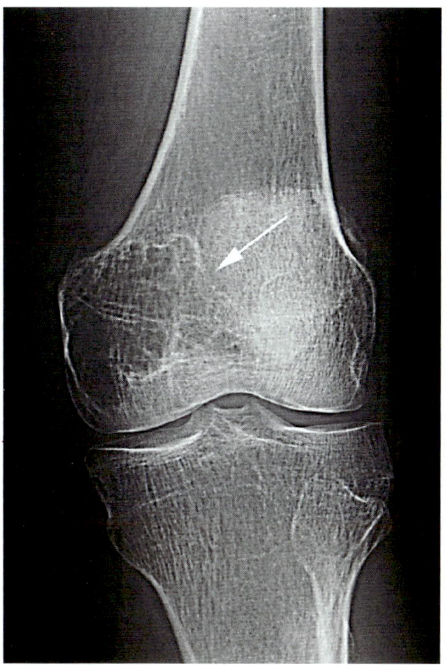

Fig. 24. Plain radiograph of the left knee. There is a relatively well defined osteolytic lesion in the medial femoral condyle that in part is surrounded by a thin sclerotic rim (arrow). The sclerotic rim indicates a slowly growing lesion (i.e. a benign lesion). However, as there is no sclerotic rim around part of the lesion, a diagnosis of benignity is put in doubt. The nature of the lesion is thus indeterminate.

Comments
In this case, the clinical data (age, site), the radiological investigation and the cytological features including immunocytochemistry were all in accordance.

Case Report 2

The patient was a middle-aged woman with a palpable tumour in the medial part of the distal left thigh.

On radiology (fig. 24), a plain radiograph of the left knee showed a relatively well defined osteolytic lesion in the medial femoral condyle, which is in part surrounded by a thin sclerotic rim (arrow in the figure). The sclerotic rim indicated a slowly growing lesion (i.e. a benign lesion), but focally there was no sclerotic rim, which made a diagnosis of benignity doubtful. Thus, the nature of the lesion was indeterminate.

FNA of the palpable tumour in the medial femoral condyle was performed by the cytopathologist. Figure 25a (MGG, low magnification) shows clustered and dispersed tumour cells mixed with osteoclast-like giant cells. In figure 25b (HE, high magnification) it can be seen that the tumour cells were large with abundant cytoplasm. The nuclei were eccentric and a faintly outlined cytoplasmic Hof was present in some cells (arrow).

A preliminary cytological diagnosis of osteosarcoma was rendered.

In Figure 25c (cytospin preparation, ALP staining, medium magnification) the tumour cells appear strongly positive for ALP.

Part of the aspirate was saved for static DNA ploidy analysis which showed an aneuploid cell population confirming malignancy.

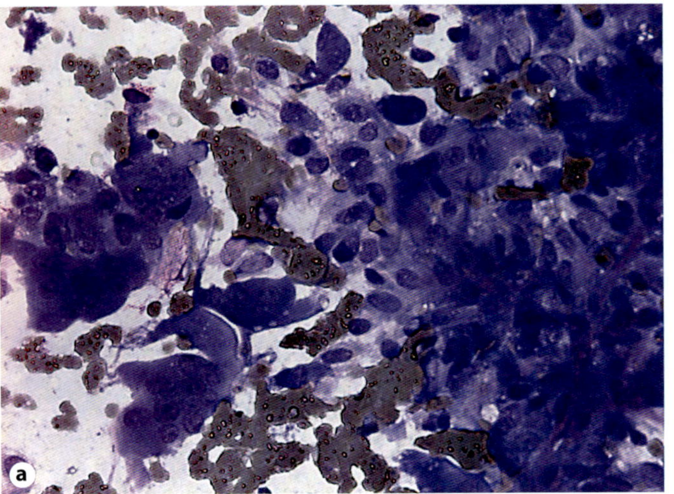

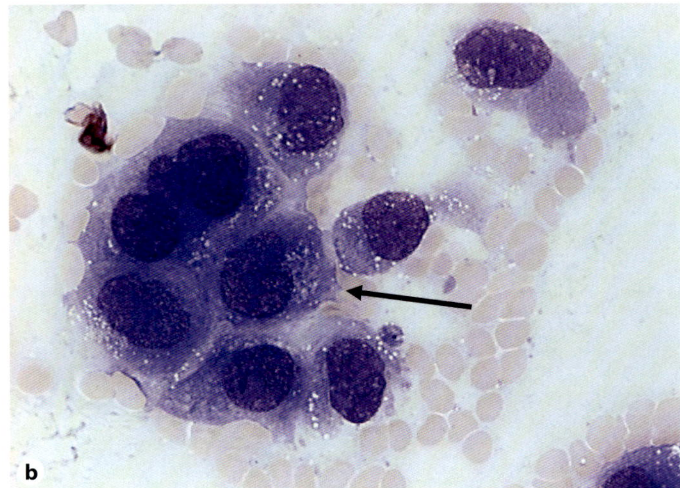

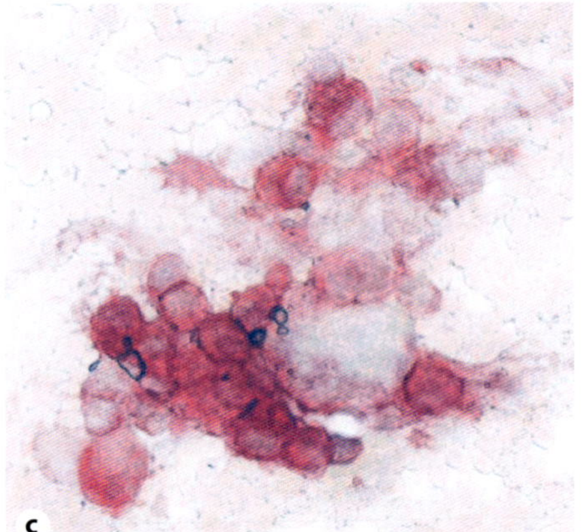

Fig. 25. **a** Clustered and dispersed tumour cells mixed with osteoclast-like giant cells. MGG, low magnification. **b** The tumour cells are large with abundant cytoplasm. The nuclei are eccentric and in some cells a faintly outlined cytoplasmic Hof is present (arrow). HE, high magnification. **c** The tumour cells are strongly positive for ALP. Cytospin preparation, ALP staining, medium magnification.

The final cytological diagnosis was giant-cell-rich osteoblastic osteosarcoma. Primary surgery was performed. The histological diagnosis was of an osteoclast-rich osteoblastic and chondroblastic osteosarcoma.

Comments

The radiological findings were inconclusive with regard to benignity or malignancy. Clinically, in view of the patient's age, carcinoma metastasis or solitary plasmacytoma were the initially favoured diagnoses. The numerous osteoclast-like giant cells together with another malignant cellular population including osteoblast-like tumour cells suggested an osteosarcoma. The diagnosis was confirmed by the strong positive ALP staining. The chondroblastic component was not represented in the FNA sample.

Chapter 6

Cytological Features of Bone Tumours in FNA Smears II: Cartilaginous Tumours

Chondroma

Chondromas are benign tumours of hyaline cartilage. The enchondromas are tumours of the medullary bone while periosteal (juxtacortical) chondromas arise from the periosteum. Enchondromas are common bone tumours with a wide age distribution, although the majority of patients are 20–40 years of age. Almost 50% of surgically removed enchondromas occur in the small bones of the hands and feet. The second commonest sites are the proximal part of the humerus and the proximal and distal femur. Enchondromas of the hands and feet are typically palpable and sometimes painful tumours. However, these tumours are commonly first discovered when a mild to moderate trauma causes a fracture. Multiple enchondromas are designated as enchondromatosis or Ollier's disease. Periosteal chondromas are less common than enchondromas and are most common in the long bones.

Radiology

See figure 26. Enchondromas are well circumscribed, often with a lobulated contour, cortical expansion and endosteal erosions. There are varying degrees of calcifications within the lesion. The radiologic characteristics of solitary and multiple lesions (Ollier's disease) are the same, although multiple lesions are often more expansile.

Periosteal or juxtacortical chondromas are characterized by a soft tissue component with erosion and periosteitis of the adjacent cortical bone. There are often calcifications within the soft tissue component.

Histopathology

Chondromas are rather paucicellular tumours with abundant hyaline cartilaginous matrix. The chondrocytes are present within lacunae, have small nuclei and sometimes small nucleoli. The chondrocytes can be arranged in small clusters or are evenly distributed. Binucleated chondrocytes may occur. Typically, chondromas of the hands and feet are more cellular and may exhibit cellular pleomorphism with relatively marked anisokaryosis.

Cytological Features

See figure 27. There are cartilaginous tissue fragments, which appear red-purple in MGG and DiffQuick and pale, faintly pink, in wet-fixed smears. Cells are in lacunae within fragments and single cells are very uncommon. The chondrocytes appear small and uniform. Chondromas of the hands and feet may be cellular and show more or less marked anisokaryosis and binucleation.

Differential Diagnosis

The differential diagnosis is low-grade malignant chondrosarcoma.

Comments

Combined evaluation of radiological and cytological features is mandatory in order to avoid a false-positive diagnosis of low-grade malignant chondrosarcoma. This is especially important in tumours of the hands and feet. It is unwise to suggest a diagnosis of chondrosarcoma even in tumours with marked cellular pleomorphism when radiologic features are unequivocally in favour of chondroma. The cytological features of chondroma have been investigated in single publications [42, 43]

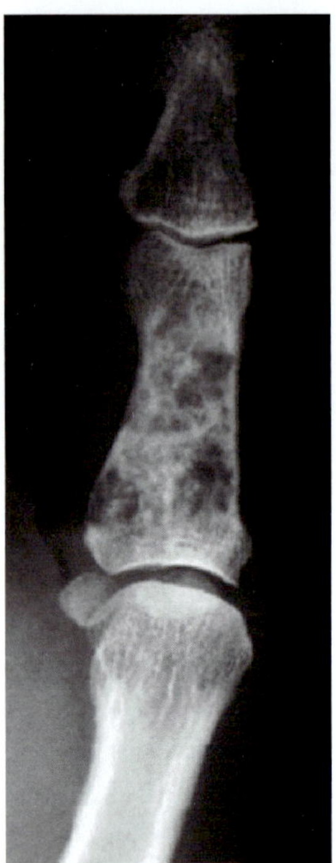

Fig. 26. Chondroma. Radiological features. PA radiograph of a finger with an enchondroma of the middle phalanx. The structure is mixed with lytic and sclerotic components. In the lytic areas there are several calcifications, which is typical of chondromatous tumours.

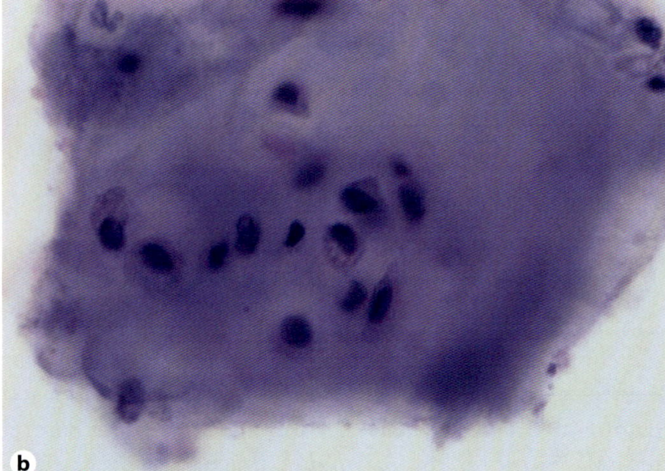

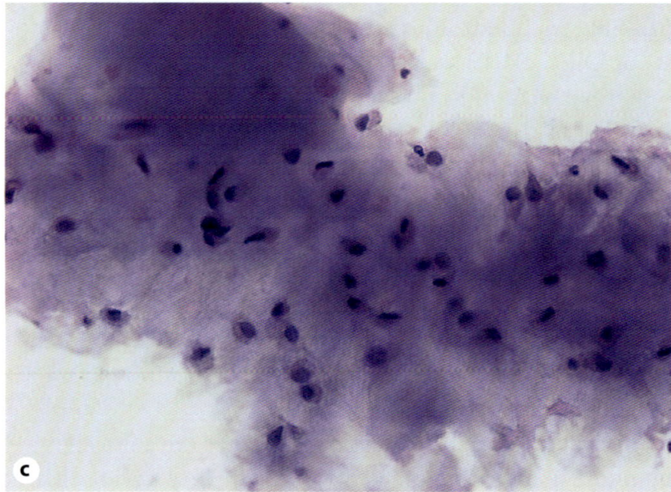

Fig. 27. Cartilaginous fragments from a chondroma of a finger. Uniform chondrocytes are situated at random in the fragments. Some chondrocytes are seen in lacunae. HE, medium magnification.

Chondroblastoma

These are rare bone tumours (<1% of bone tumours), predominantly occurring in children and young adults. The peak incidence is in the second decade. More than three quarters of chondroblastomas occur in the epiphyseal regions of the long tubular bones. Unusual sites are calcaneus, talus, patella and the temporal bone. Many patients complain of pain, often mild, sometimes for many years.

Radiology
See figure 28. Chondroblastomas are usually well demarcated lytic lesions with a thin sclerotic rim. Sometimes small calcifications are seen within the lytic lesion, and in those instances the radiological image is diagnostic.

Histopathology
Chondroblastoma cells are uniform, rounded to polygonal with well defined cell borders and rounded or ovoid nuclei. The nuclei often display grooves or clefts and contain small nucleoli. Some nuclei can be large and hyperchromatic. The cytoplasm is clear or faintly eosiniphilic. Mitoses are often

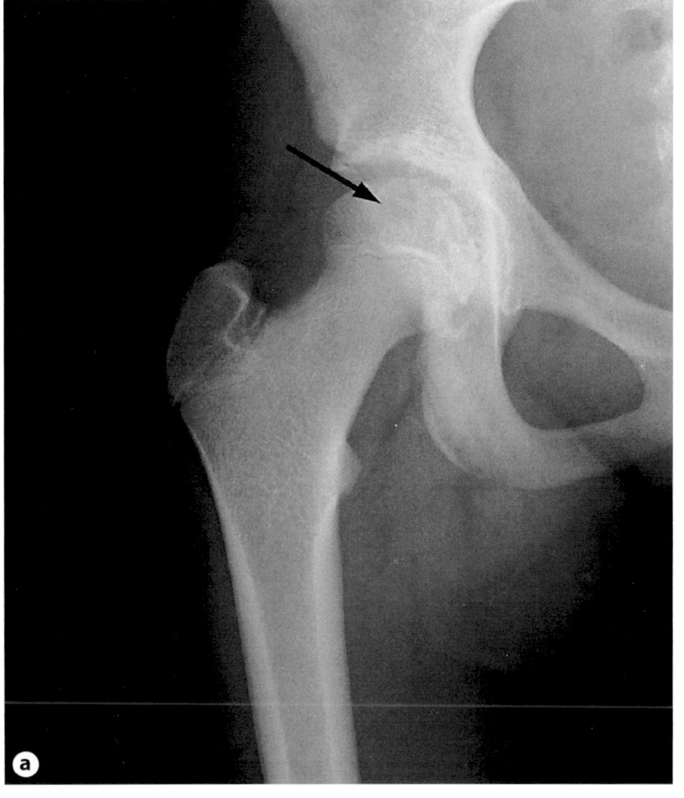

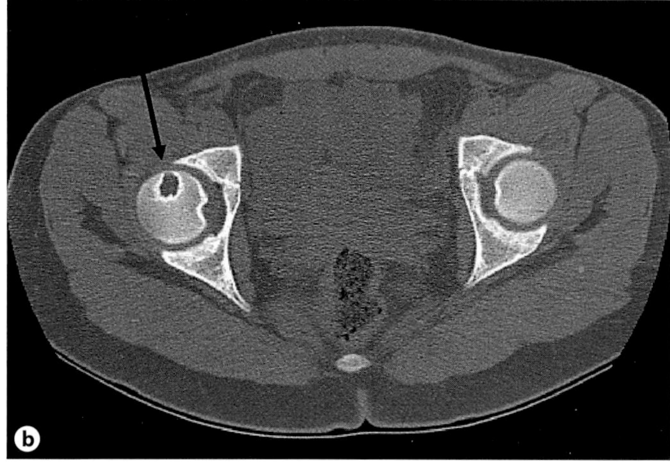

Fig. 28. Chondroblastoma. Radiologic features. **a** AP radiograph of the right hip. A small lytic lesion can be identified in the epiphysis of the femur (arrow). **b** Axial CT of the hip joints of the same patient. On the right side, a well demarcated lytic lesion surrounded by thin sclerotic margins is seen in the femoral epiphysis (arrow).

observed. The chondroblasts are arranged in sheets containing numerous randomly distributed giant cells of osteoclastic type. There is a varying amount of chondroid matrix. A typical find is a network of pericellular calcifications.

Cytological Features

See figure 29. There are fragments of chondroid matrix and multinucleated giant cells of osteoclastic type are also seen. Mononuclear cells are rounded with well defined borders and rounded nuclei with fine chromatin and small nucleoli. The nuclei are often indented or lobulated or exhibit longitudinal grooves. Slight anisokaryosis and binucleation may be found. There may rarely be small calcifications.

Differential Diagnosis

The differential diagnoses are: chondromyxoid fibroma; giant cell tumour; aneurysmal bone cyst, and clear-cell chondrosarcoma.

Comments

The cytology of chondroblastoma has been described in 4 series [42, 44–46]. As in our own experience, the most common cytological feature was chondroblasts with indented, lobulated or grooved nuclei. Another clue to the diagnosis is the presence of chondroid matrix and osteoclast-like giant cells. According to Kilpatrick et al. [46], the presence of typical chondroblasts in an epiphyseal bone tumour with classic radiographic features of chondroblastoma is sufficient to suggest the diagnosis even without matrix fragments and giant cells. The mono- and binucleated stromal cells of a giant-cell tumour are smaller, with smaller rounded nuclei, and chondroid fragments are not typical.

Chondromyxoid fibroma occurs in the same age group as chondroblastoma but is situated in the metaphysis. Aneurysmal bone cyst-like areas may be found in chondroblastoma and in those cases the radiological features may be interpreted as an aneurysmal bone cyst. However, cytologically these combined lesions have no malignant features and are diagnosed as benign bone tumours with numerous giant cells. The cytological appearance of clear-cell chondrosarcoma in FNA smears is not sufficiently defined, but in histological sections the large tumour cells with clear cytoplasm are evidently malignant.

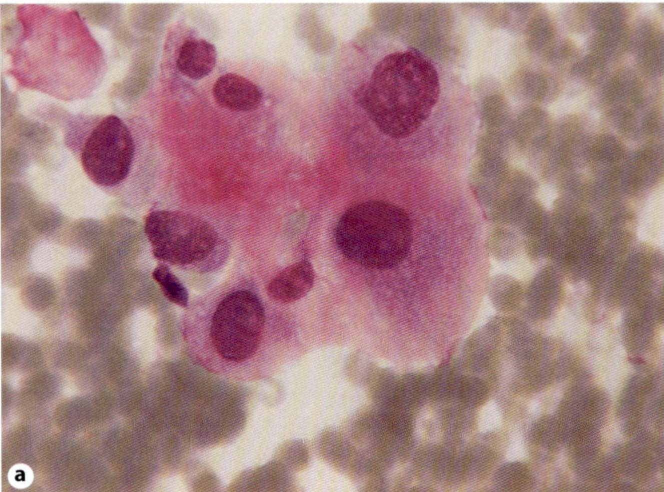

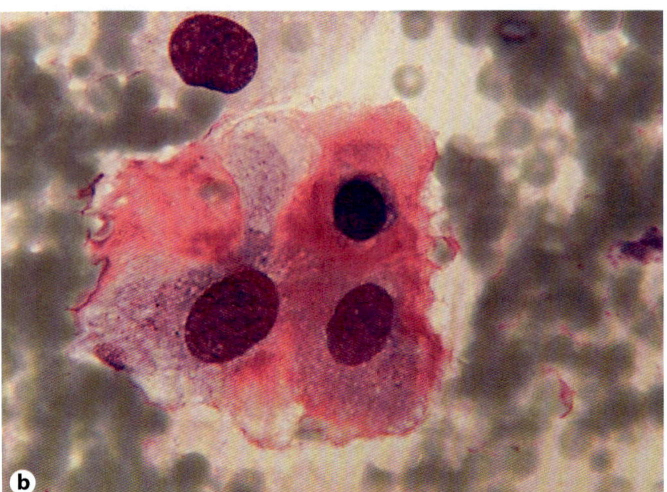

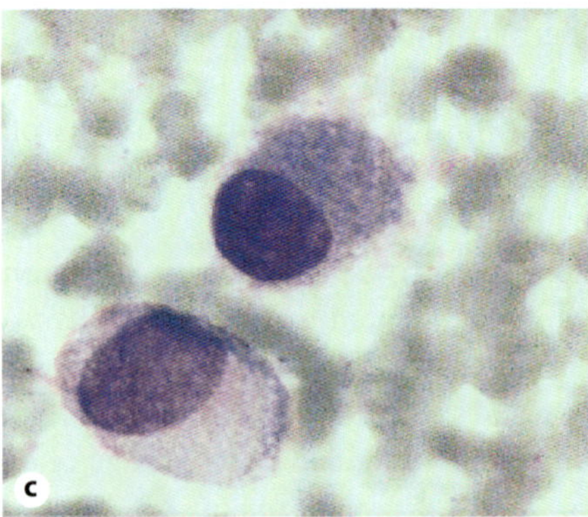

Fig. 29. **a**, **b** Mononuclear rounded cells are seen within fragments of chondroid matrix. A few dispersed cells with rather abundant well defined cytoplasm are present. MGG, medium magnification. **c** Dispersed chondroblastoma cells with well defined cytoplasm and rounded nuclei. MGG, high magnification.

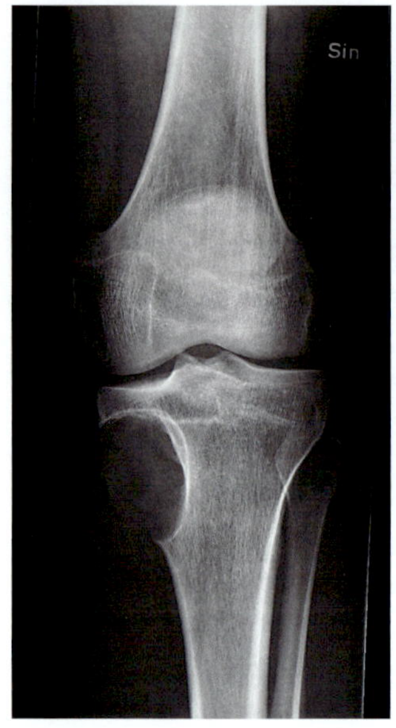

Fig. 30. Chondromyxoid fibroma. Radiologic features. AP radiograph of the left knee. A well defined lytic lesion with thin sclerotic margins is seen in the proximal tibia.

Chondromyxoid Fibroma

Chondromyxoid fibroma is very uncommon, comprising 1–2% of benign bone tumours and about 2% of cartilaginous tumours [30]. The most frequent sites are the femur and the tibia, other common sites are the flat bones, especially the ileum. Most tumours appear in the second and third decades and are typically located in the metaphysis of the long bones.

Radiology

See figure 30. Chondromyxoid fibromas are osteolytic and eccentrically located. The lesions are elongated, vary in size and may be up to 10 cm in length. The cortex over the lesion is often expanded with endosteal sclerosis. A complete penetration of the cortex may be seen as a hemispherical osseous defect.

Histopathology

The typical chondromyxoid fibroma is a lobulated tumour with abundant myxoid background matrix. Spindly and stellate cells are embedded in the myxoid matrix and, characteristically, the tumour lobuli have hypocellular centres and hypercellular periphery. The cells often have cytoplasmic extensions and in many tumours there are single cells with large, hyperchromatic and pleomorphic nuclei. Foci of hyaline cartilage are present in some tumours and osteoclast-like giant cells may be seen at the periphery of the tumour lobules. Mitoses are rare.

Cytological Features
See figure 31. There is a myxoid background matrix. Spindle-shaped or stellate cells are dispersed or clustered. There are cartilaginous fragments and osteoclast-like giant cells.

Differential Diagnosis
The differential diagnosis is chondrosarcoma.

Comments
There are single reports of FNAC in this rare tumour [47–49] and our experience is limited to a few cases. The spindly and stellate cells vary in size and may exhibit pleomorphic nuclei with hyperchromasia and prominent nucleoli. Lacunar chondroblast-like cells in the cartilaginous fragments may also show pleomorphism and binucleation. Myxoid chondrosarcoma may be suspected in FNA smears when cartilaginous fragments are lacking and clusters of spindle cells show anisokaryosis and nuclear hyperchromasia in cases where the radiological features are not typical.

Chondrosarcoma

Chondrosarcomas are a heterogeneous group of cartilaginous malignant tumours. The vast majority of the so-called primary conventional chondrosarcomas are intramedullary tumours. Primary periosteal (juxtacortical) chondrosarcoma is very rare. The term secondary chondrosarcoma is reserved for those tumours which arise in patients with Ollier's disease and Mafucci syndrome. Special variants of chondrosarcoma include dedifferentiated, mesenchymal and clear-cell tumours. Roughly 90% of chondrosarcomas are primary conventional. They are the second most common of the primary bone sarcomas, up to 27% of primary bone sarcomas are chondrosarcomas in the published series. Primary chondrosarcoma is rare before the age of 45, and most appear in patients between 50 and 80 years of age. The most common sites are the pelvic bones and the extremities. Rare sites include spine, craniofascial bones and the small bones of the hands and feet.

Radiology
See figure 32. Conventional chondrosarcomas are often located intramedullarly in the metaphyses of long bones, especially in the femur and humerus. The tumours are

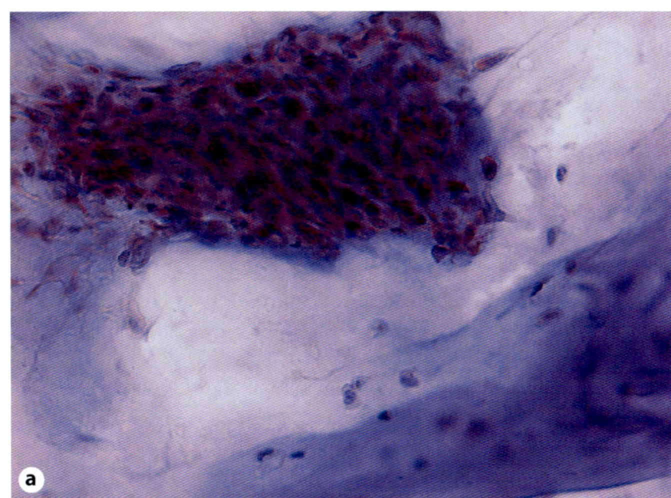

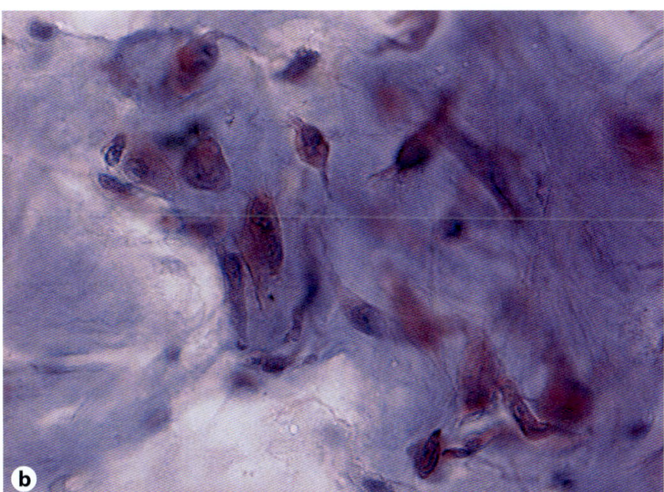

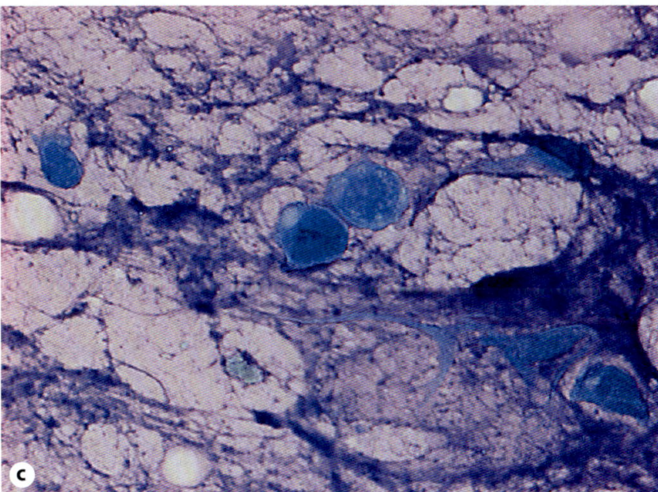

Fig. 31. a Clustered spindly or stellate cells in a myxoid background. HE, medium magnification. **b** The spindly and stellate cells exhibit moderate anisokaryosis. HE, high magnification. **c** Chondroblast-like cells in the myxoid background show moderate pleomorphism. MGG, high magnification.

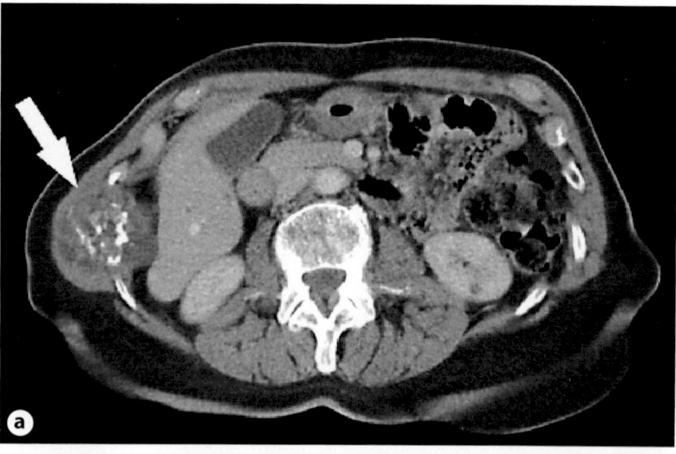

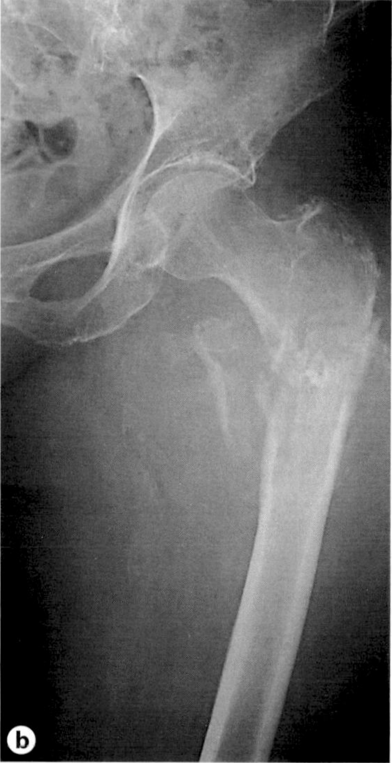

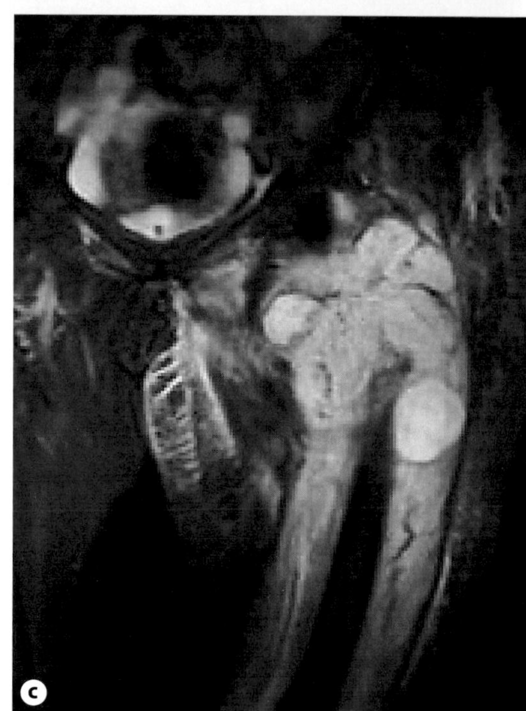

Fig. 32. Chondrosarcoma. Radiological features. **a** Chondrosarcoma of a rib on the right side. Highly expansive lesion with several intralesional calcifications (arrow). **b** AP radiograph of the proximal left femur. There is a pathological intertrochanteric fracture with avulsion of the lesser trochanter. There is general sclerosis at the level of the fracture, but no obvious bone destruction. **c** T2-weighted fat-saturated coronal MRI section of the same lesion as **b**. There is an extensive soft tissue component with high signal intensity.

elongated and often exhibit a lytic erosion of the endosteum of the bone. In the typical case there are intratumoral calcifications. When these calcifications have a regular shape a low-grade malignant chondrosarcoma is the rule. The same pattern of calcifications and lytic lesions may be present in benign enchondromas in the same site. Radiologically they can not be distinguished from low-grade chondrosarcoma. The only sign of differential diagnostic value is whether the lesion is painful, which may happen in chondrosarcoma, but not in benign enchondroma, with the exception of the enchondromas of hands and feet.

In high grade chondrosarcoma the tumour displays a more moth-eaten and permeative pattern. A soft tissue component may be present in cases with permeative growth with cortical destruction. This pattern is not seen in purely central chondrosarcomas.

It is often difficult to radiologically differentiate a benign chondroma from one with malignant transformation. In the malignant cases the cartilagionous cap is often bulky. CT may be of help to distinguish benign from malignant tumours of this kind.

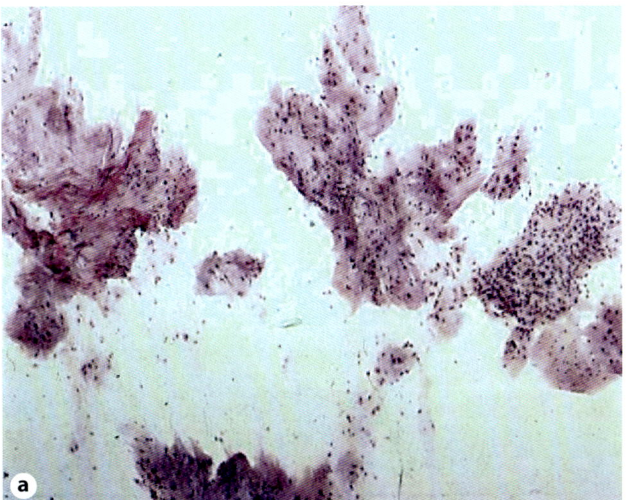

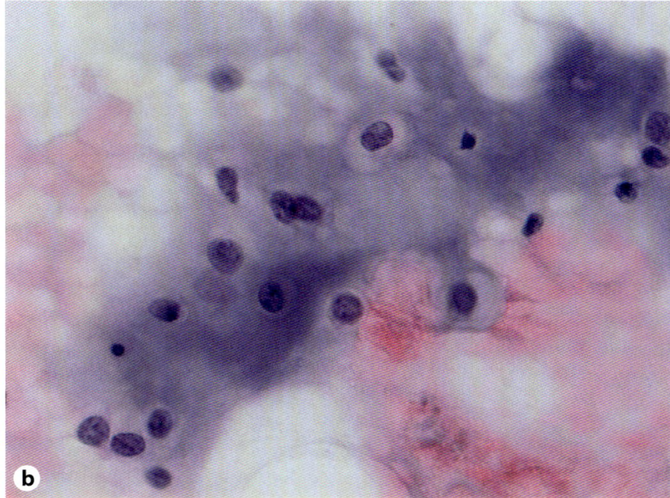

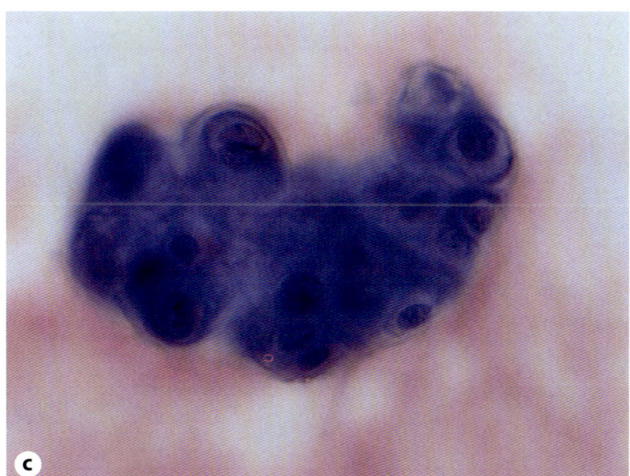

Fig. 33. Low-grade chondrosarcoma (grades 1 and 2). **a** Fragments of hyaline cartilage. Note the variable cellularity of the fragments. HE, low magnification. **b** A hyaline cartilaginous fragment with rather uniform tumour cells in lacunae. HE, medium magnification. **c** This tumour fragment is cellular. The nuclear atypia is still slight to moderate. HE, high magnification.

Histopathology

Primary chondrosarcomas are lobulated tumours. The cartilaginous lobules are of varying size and may show varying degrees of myxoid change and calcification. Compared to chondromas, chondrosarcomas are more cellular tumours, although the cellularity varies from one area to another. The atypia of the malignant chondrocytes is variable. Binucleated tumour cells are often seen. Malignancy grading is important in primary chondrosarcoma with regard to prognosis. In the grading system recommended, chondrosarcomas are graded on a scale of 1–3 [2, 30]. Grade 1 tumours are moderately cellular with minimal or slight atypia and cytologically resemble chondromas. Grade 2 tumours are more cellular and the cellular and nuclear atypia (anisokaryosis, hyperchromasia, enlarged nucleoli) is more marked. Binucleated cells are not uncommon and areas of myxoid change frequent. Grade 3 chondrosarcomas display prominent atypia and are highly cellular, mitoses are easily found, the tumour cells are markedly atypical and there is abundant myxoid change. Grade 3 chondrosarcomas are rare tumours. Chondrosarcoma of grades 1 and 2 are considered low-grade malignant, grade 3 as high grade.

Cytological Features

Grade 1 and 2 tumours (low-grade): See figure 33. Fragments of hyaline cartilage of variable size appear and have variable cellularity. There is a myxoid background matrix. Single cells are infrequent. Mono- and binucleated rounded cells with well defined cytoplasm are seen, often in lacunae. Threre is slight to moderate cellular atypia and rarely mitoses.

Grade 3 tumours (high-grade): See figure 34. There is an abundant myxoid background matrix and relatively few fragments of hyaline cartilage, which are often highly cellular. Many dispersed tumour cells are seen. There is marked

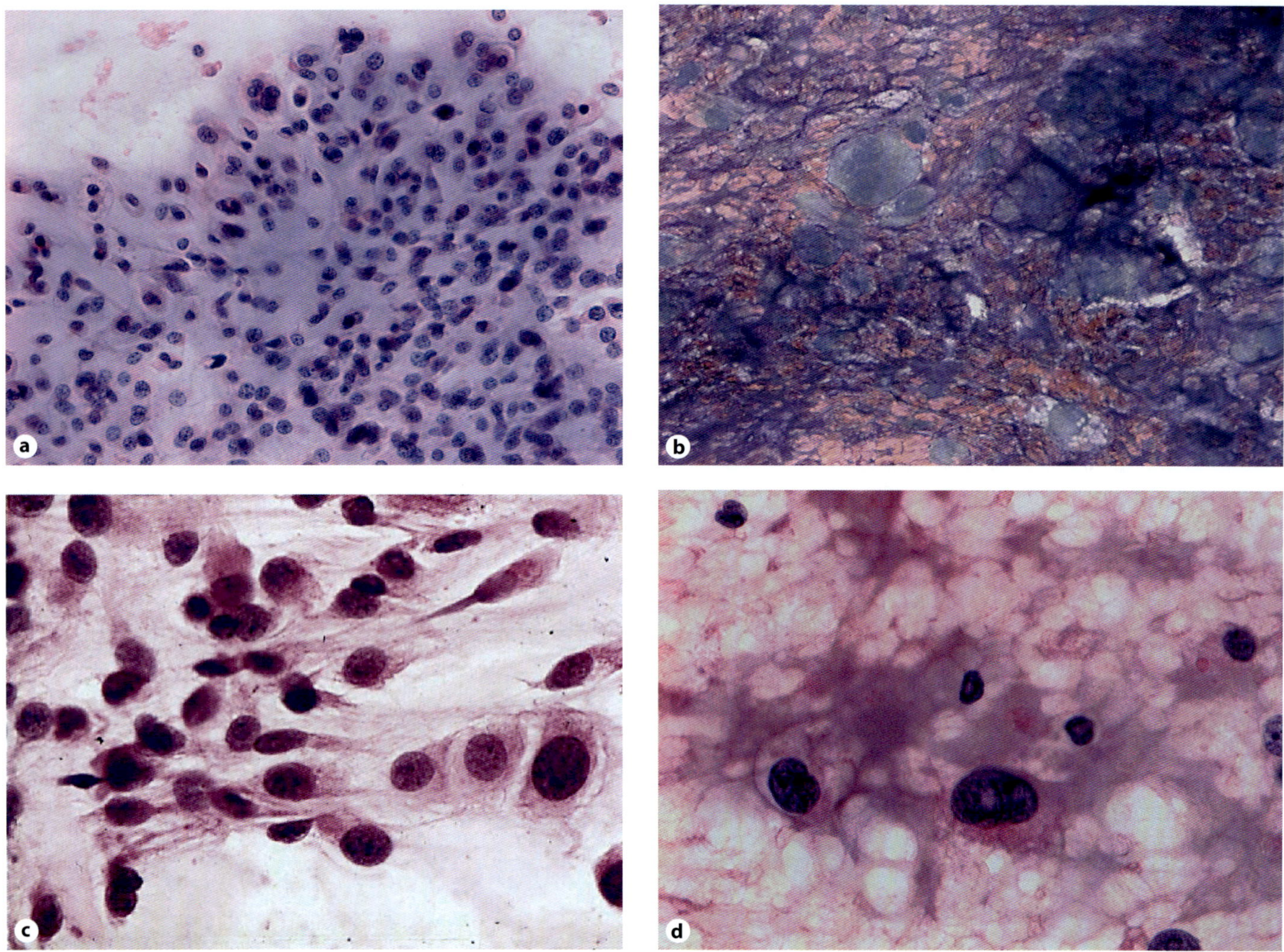

Fig. 34. High-grade chondrosarcoma (grade 3). **a** Compared to low-grade chondrosarcoma, the tumour fragments are highly cellular. HE, low magnification. **b** Abundant myxoid background matrix obscuring the nuclear details in MGG is often present. MGG, medium magnification. **c** Compared to low-grade chondrosarcoma (grades 1 and 2), tumour fragments are often scant in the smears and the fragments are generally highly cellular. HE, medium magnification. **d** Compared to low-grade chondrosarcoma there is marked cellular and nuclear atypia. HE, medium magnification.

cellular and nuclear pleomorphism with prominent nucleoli and occasional mitosis.

Differential Diagnosis

The differential diangnoses are: chondroma; chondroblastic osteosarcoma; chordoma, and metastastatic adenocarcinoma.

Comments

Most primary chondrosarcomas are easy to needle and the yield is often surprisingly high. Chondrosarcoma with reactive periosteal bone formation and heavily calcified tumours are exceptions. The cytology of primary chondrosarcoma has been relatively thoroughly described in the cytological literature [15, 42, 50–53]. The most important diagnostic features common to all published series are the presence of hyaline cartilaginous fragments together with a myxoid background matrix. Cartilaginous fragments and matrix stain strongly red/blue and violet in MGG and DiffQuick and pale pink in HE. The strong staining in air-dried preparations makes the study of cellular and nuclear details much more difficult than in HE or Pap-stained smears. On the other hand the matrix stains poorly in wet-fixed material. Preparation of wet-fixed as well as air-dried smears is strongly recommended when a cartilaginous tumour is suspected.

Another diagnostic feature emphasized in all cited publications is the relation between cartilaginous fragments and myxoid background matrix. Fragments dominate in low-grade chondrosarcoma, especially grade 1 tumours, while the presence of both fragments and matrix is typical for grade 2 tumours. Abundant myxoid matrix and very few cartilaginous fragments are the characteristic findings in smears from high-grade (grade 3) chondrosarcoma. The accuracy of grading of chondrosarcoma in FNA-material has been investigated by Lerma et al. [51]. Concordance with histological grade was high in grade 2 and 3 tumours in the evaluated series. Low-grade, especially grade 1, chondrosarcoma may be difficult to distinguish from chordoma in biopsy samples and the same pitfall applies to FNA. Clinical and radiological features are important in the diagnostic evaluation. This is especially the case of cartilaginous tumours in the small bones of the hands and feet. Chondromas in these sites may exhibit rather marked cellular pleomorphism in FNA smears, as previously stated. However, chondrosarcoma in these sites are very rare. From the clinical point of view, it is not a serious problem. In a retrospective analysis of the behaviour of low-grade chondrosarcoma, Bauer et al. [53] demonstrated a similar long-term prognosis as regards recurrence rates and metastatic potential in 40 enchondromas and 40 low-grade chondrosarcomas. They concluded that the distinction between these tumours was of little clinical significance. The problem to distinguish chondroblastic osteosarcoma from high-grade chondrosarcoma is addressed in the comments on osteosarcoma diagnosis.

When dealing with tumours in the vertebrae and sacrum, chordoma may be a problem for the differential diagnosis. The structure of the myxoid matrix of chordoma is, however, different from that in chondrosarcoma. It is typically fibrillar and forms a network of thin strands encircling individual cells, singly or in groups. Furthermore the large, cytoplasm-rich and vacuolated cells with central nuclei, corresponding to physaliferous cells are present in every case of chordoma and are not part of the cellular spectrum of chondrosarcoma.

The single cells in smears from grade 3 chondrosarcoma may have an epithelioid appearance and may be mistaken for adenocarcinoma cells in wet-fixed preparations where the myxoid matrix stains only faintly.

Immunocytochemistry is of help in the differential diagnosis between chondrosarcoma and chordoma. Although both tumours stain positively with S-100 protein, chordoma cells are positive with EMA as well as low-molecular-weight keratins. Immunocytochemistry is also of diagnostic help in the distinction between high-grade (grade 3) chondrosarcoma and metastatic adenocarcinoma.

DNA ploidy analysis of chondrosarcoma can be helpful when the cytological evaluation is inconclusive regarding benignity or malignancy. High-grade chondrosarcomas are often non-diploid [21, 22]. Our unpublished observations of flow cytometric and static cytometric analyses of chondrosarcoma aspirates correspond well with the cited reports. Thus, a non-diploid histogram strongly favours chondrosarcoma.

Dedifferentiated Chondrosarcoma

Dedifferentiated chondrosarcoma is a distinct subtype of chondrosarcoma with 2 defined components: a low-grade chondrosarcoma or chondroma and a high-grade malignant non-cartilaginous sarcoma. There is a distinct transition between the 2 tumour components. Approximately 10% of all chondrosarcomas belong to this category. The most frequent bones involved are the femur, the pelvic bones and humerus.

Radiology

Radiologically these tumours have a moth-eaten pattern. One area is devoid of intratumoral calcifications with signs of more aggressive bone destruction, at times with penetration of the cortical bone and a soft tissue component. The radiological clue to the diagnosis is the co-existence of the 2 types of tumour destruction in the same lesion.

Histopathology

As stated above, the cartilaginous part is most often a low-grade chondrosarcoma. The high-grade non-cartilaginous sarcoma is most frequently a pleomorphic sarcoma of malignant fibrous histiocytoma type but osteosarcoma, rhabdomyosarcoma and spindle-cell sarcoma have also been described.

Cytological Features

See figure 35. The cytological features of low-grade (grades 1–2) chondrosarcoma, as described above, are combined in the same sample with features of high-grade malignant sarcoma, most often similar to pleomorphic soft tissue sarcoma of the malignant fibrous histiocytoma type. Infrequently there are cytological features of osteosarcoma or rhabdomyosarcoma.

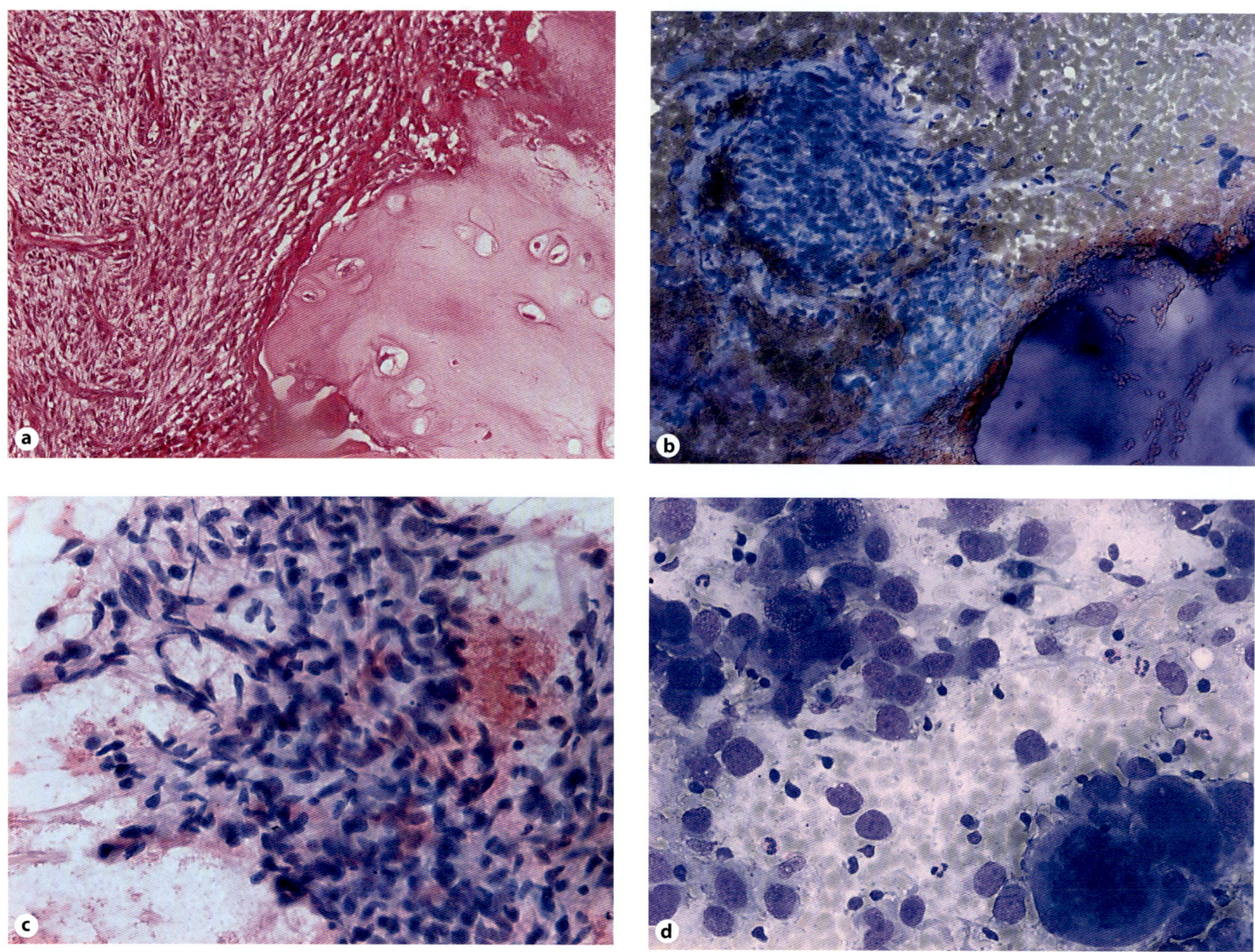

Fig. 35. Dedifferentiated chondrosarcoma. **a** The 2 tissue components necessary for the diagnosis are present in this histologic field of view. Part of a low-grade chondrosarcoma is seen in the lower right corner. There is a distinct transition to a highly cellular, high-grade spindle cell sarcoma in the upper left part. HE, low magnification. **b** Part of the FNA smear from the same case showing part of a paucicellular hyaline cartilage fragment in the lower right corner. To the left are tight clusters of spindle cells. MGG, low magnification. **c** The spindle-cell population is atypical showing anisokaryosis and hyperchromasia. HE, medium magnification.) **d** Smear from another dedifferentiated chondrosarcoma. The pattern is of a high-grade pleomorphic sarcoma resembling an osteosarcoma. MGG, medium magnification.

Differential Diagnosis

The differential diagnoses are: osteosarcoma; pleomorphic high grade soft tissue sarcoma, and rhabdomyosarcoma.

Comments

The clue to the diagnosis is the double cell population in aspirates from the same tumour.

The cytology of dedifferentiated chondrosarcoma is incompletely described. In one published case the high-grade malignant component was a pleomorphic sarcoma [54]. One single case from our file displayed signs of a high-grade malignant spindle-cell sarcoma combined with a chondrosarcoma component. Rinas et al. [55] have highlighted potential sampling error as a diagnostic pitfall, emphasizing the importance of clinical and radiological correlation when only 1 tissue component is present in the samples. Positive ALP staining favours osteosarcoma as the sarcomatous component. Immunocytochemistry may be of help to identify rhabdomyosarcoma.

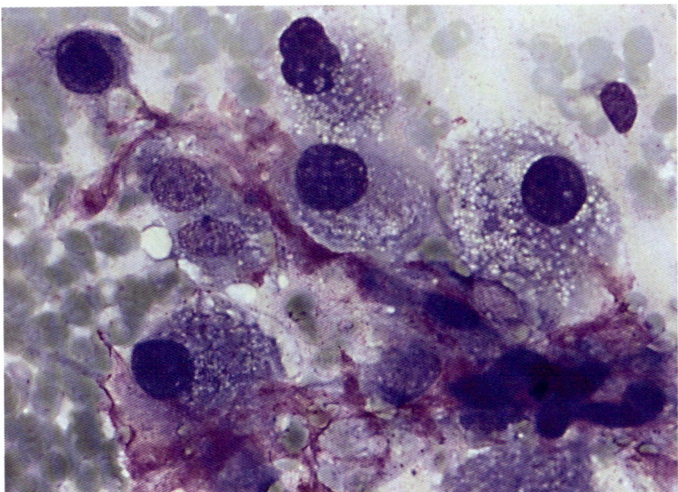

Fig. 36. Clear-cell chondrosarcoma. A group of large cells with abundant clear cytoplasm and round to oval nuclei are embedded in a faintly stained chondroid background matrix. MGG, high magnification.

Clear-Cell Chondrosarcoma

Clear-cell chondrosarcoma is an infrequent variant of low-grade chondrosarcoma, which most often arises in the epiphyses of the humerus and the femur.

Radiology
These tumours are osteolytic, often with well demarcated margins with or without a sclerotic rim. Calcifications are often present. Radiographically, clear-cell chondrosarcoma may be impossible to differentiate from chondroblastoma.

Histopathology
The typical tumour cells have a clear or pale pink cytoplasm and central nuclei. Some cells resemble chondroblasts. Many tumours also contain areas of conventional low-grade chondrosarcoma. Spiculae of woven bone may be found together with the clear-cell component, as may osteoclast-like giant cells.

Cytological Features
See figure 36. Small cartilaginous fragments are found in a background of myxoid matrix. Large (epithelioid) tumour cells have well demarcated, abundant vacuolated cytoplasm and hyperchromatic nuclei with central nucleoli. There are occasional osteoclast-like giant cells.

Differential Diagnosis
The differential diagnoses are chondroblastoma and metastatic adenocarcinoma.

Comments
Only single cases of clear-cell chondrosarcoma have been reported [42]. The most important diagnostic problem is clear-cell chondrosarcoma versus chondroblastoma. The tumour cells in clear-cell chondrosarcoma are generally more consistently atypical, with hyperchromasia and prominent nucleoli, and they lack nuclear grooves.

Immunocytochemical staining is of help to exclude or confirm adenocarcinoma. The cells of clear-cell chondrosarcoma are strongly S-100 protein positive and keratin-negative.

Mesenchymal Chondrosarcoma

Mesenchymal chondrosarcoma is a rare tumour with a bimorphic pattern, composed of islands of hyaline cartilage and a malignant small round cell population. Most cases occur in the second and third decades. The craniofacial bones (jawbones), ribs, vertebrae and the ilium are the most common sites.

Radiology
The radiological signs of mesenchymal chondrosarcoma are the same as of conventional chondrosarcoma (a tumour with a permeative growth pattern, intralesional calcifications and periosteitis). A soft tissue component, often with stippled calcifications, is not uncommon. The only clue to suggest a mesenchymal chondrosarcoma is the relative young age of the patients.

Histopathology
Islands of hyaline cartilage are mixed with sheets of undifferentiated small rounded cells resembling the tumour cells of conventional Ewing's sarcoma. A haemangiopericytomatous vascular pattern is common.

Cytological Features
See figure 37. Cellular aspirates. There are clusters of small malignant cells with sparse cytoplasm and rounded, ovoid or sometimes elongated nuclei. Coarse nuclear chromatin and small nucleoli are seen. There is variable presence of fibrillar myxoid matrix associated with the cell clusters and also variable presence of fragments of hyaline cartilage.

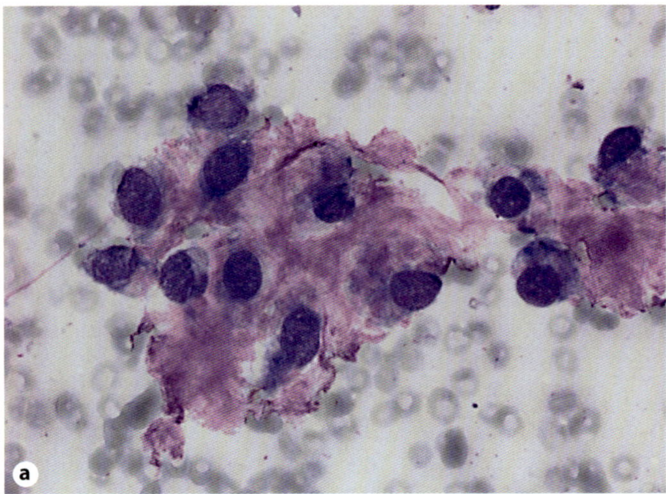

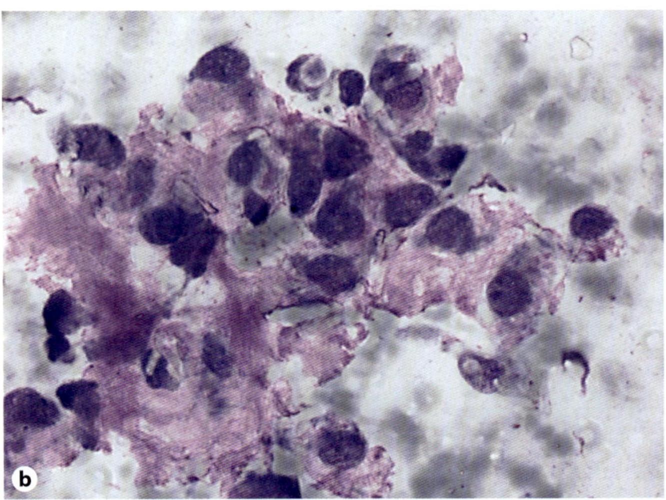

Fig. 37. a, b Mesenchymal chondrosarcoma. Clusters of relatively small tumour cells with sparse cytoplasm and irregular nuclei. The cells are embedded in a blue-violet myxoid matrix. MGG, high magnification.

Differential Diagnosis

The differential diagnoses are: Ewing's sarcoma; small-cell osteosarcoma; embryonal rhabdomyosarcoma, and non-Hodgkin lymphoma.

Comments

Very few cases of mesenchymal chondrosarcoma have been reported in the cytological literature [42]. When a biphasic pattern (cartilaginous fragments and small malignant cells) is not obvious and only a small malignant cell population is present, the differential diagnosis versus other small-cell malignancies is very difficult and ancillary techniques are necessary for a correct diagnosis.

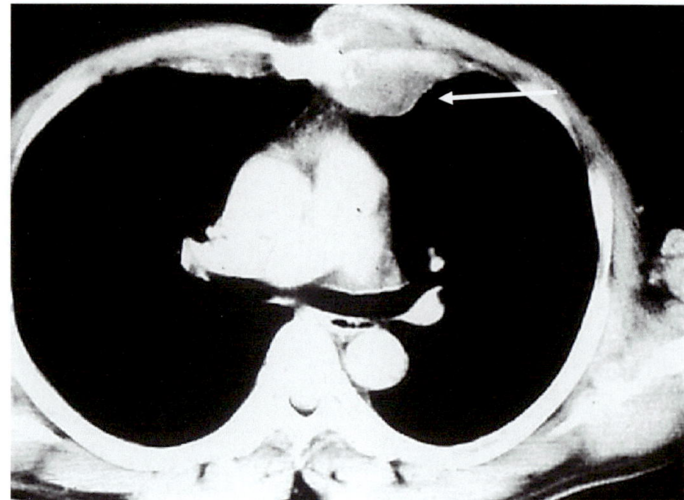

Fig. 38. Radiological features. CT of the chest with the patient in a supine position. Bony destruction of a left-sided rib, close to the sternum. Tumour expansion anteriorly and posteriorly with calcifications in the soft tissue component, indicating a malignant chondromatous tumour (a chondrosarcoma).

The typical immunophenotype of mesenchymal chondrosarcoma is S-100 protein positivity in the cartilaginous areas and CD56 and C99 positivity in the small-cell population. This immunoprofile makes differentiation from Ewing's sarcoma difficult in cases without cartilaginous fragments. Small cell osteosarcoma is another diagnostic problem. Small-cell osteosarcoma may exhibit CD99 membrane positivity in some cases but stains positively for osteonectin and osteocalcin. A rather broad panel of antibodies is necessary when only the small-cell population is present, including FLI-1, desmin, CD45, CD20, CD3, CD10, TdT and osteocalcin and osteonectin.

The 11;22 translocation, typical for the Ewing family of tumours is not considered to appear in mesenchymal chondrosarcoma [30].

Case Report 3

The patient was a middle-aged male who was referred to the Musculoskeletal Tumour Centre because of a 3 cm large, firm, immobile tumour to the left of the sternal bone.

The radiological examination was a CT of the chest with the patient in supine position (fig. 38). Bony destruction of a rib close to the left side of the sternum. Tumour expansion ventrally and dorsally, with calcifications within the soft tissue component, indicating a malignant chondromatous tumour, i.e. a chondrosarcoma.

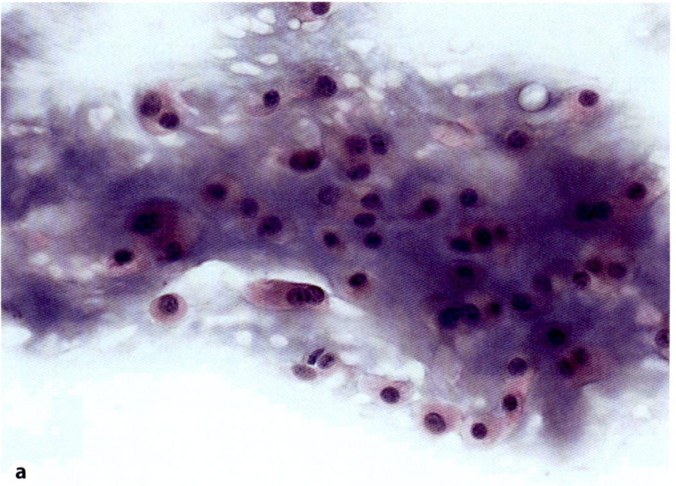

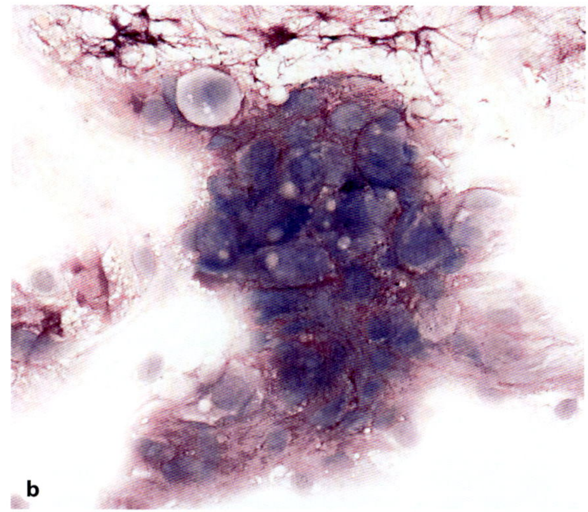

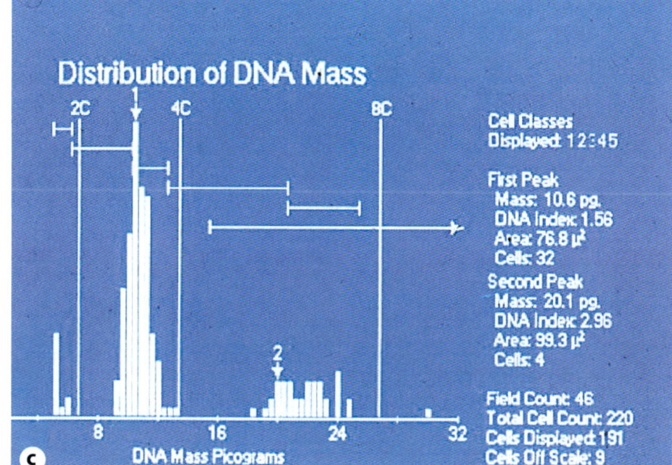

Fig. 39. a A fragment of fairly cellular hyaline chondromatous tumour tissue. Irregularly distributed atypical chondrocytes, many of them binucleated. HE, low magnification. **b** The myxoid background matrix is very evident in the MGG stained smear, but the cellular and nuclear details are difficult to appreciate due to the strong staining. MGG, medium magnification. **c** Static DNA ploidy analysis. The histogram illustrates an evident non-diploid cellular population.

FNA was performed by the cytopathologist.

Fig. 39a (HE, low magnification) shows A fragment of rather cellular hyaline chondromatous tumour tissue. Irregularly distributed atypical chondrocytes, many of them binucleated. Fig. 39b (MGG, Medium magnification) shows the myxoid background matrix is very evident in the MGG-stained smear but due to the strong staining, the cellular and nuclear details are difficult to appreciate. One smear was saved for Feulgen-staining. In Fig. 39c (Histogram Static DNA ploidy analysis) the histogram illustrates an evident non-diploid cell population.

The cytological diagnosis was high-grade chondrosarcoma (most probably grade III).

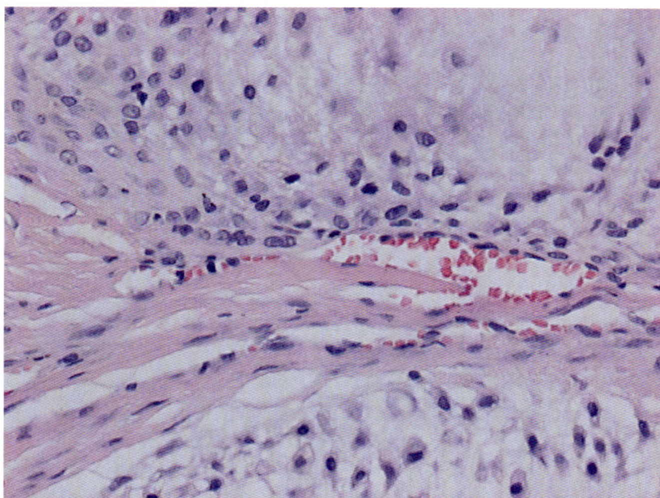

Fig. 40. A part of the resected tumour specimen. A lobulated chondromatous tumour with irregularly distributed chondrocytes with evident atypia. HE, low magnification.

Figure 40 (HE) shows part of the resected tumour specimen, a lobulated chondromatous tumour with irregularly distributed chondrocytes with evident atypia.

The final diagnosis was chondrosarcoma, malignancy grade III.

Comments

In this case, there is a concordance between the radiological and cytological features. The DNA-ploidy analysis, furthermore, strengthened the impression that the chondrosarcoma was a high-grade tumour.

Chapter 7

Cytological Features of Bone Tumours in FNA Smears III: Ewing Family Tumours

The Ewing Family of Tumours

Between 1983 and 1994 several studies clearly demonstrated that skeletal and extraskeletal classical Ewing's sarcoma, atypical Ewing's sarcoma, primitive neuroectodermal tumour (PNET), neuroepithelioma and the Askin tumour belong to the same group of small cell tumours defined by specific chimeric transcripts [56, 57]. Ewing family tumours (EFT) are considered to be neuroectodermal tumours with variable clinical presentation, variable morphology and variable ultrastructure but with a common basal immunophenotype and genotype. Classical Ewing's sarcoma (skeletal and extraskeletal) is considered as the most primitive and PNET the most differentiated in regard to neuroectodermal differentiation. PNET is relatively rare in bone, representing approximately 10% of EFT [2].

EFT is diagnosed in 6–8% of primary malignant bone tumours, which is the third most frequent primary bone sarcoma after osteosarcoma and chondrosarcoma. Approximately 80% arise in patients younger than 20 years of age, EFT is rare before the age of 5 and after the age of 30 and extremely rare in older patients. In our files going back to 1980, there is 1 patient on record aged 67.

Most common sites are the shafts of the long bones the pelvic bones, ribs and spine. EFT has, however, been diagnosed in almost every bone in the skeleton including craniofacial bones and the scapula. Extraskeletal EFT has been diagnosed in various parts of the body (cutaneous, subcutaneous, paraspinal, in the retroperitoneum, kidney and breast). More than 90% of EFT show cytoplasmic membrane positivity with CD99 and about 75% nuclear staining with the FLI-1-antibody [58, 59]. The more differentiated varieties (atypical Ewing's Sarcoma and PNET) express neuroectodermal markers, such as neuron-specific enolase, chromograninA and synaptophysin. Approximately 90% of EFT harbour the chromosomal translocation t(11;22)(q24;q12) involving the EWS gene on chromosome 22 and the FLI-1 gene on chromosome 11 resulting in the EWS/FLI-1 transcript.

Radiology
See figure 41. Classical Ewing's sarcoma is an aggressive tumour characterized by a permeative or moth-eaten growth pattern, periosteitis and a soft tissue component. The tumour is often not very well defined by conventional radiography. There is often an extensive spiculated periosteal reaction as 'hair on end' or several layers of 'onion peel' type. The tumour is, in most cases, a medullary lesion, but the signs are most prominent in the cortical bone. The soft tissue

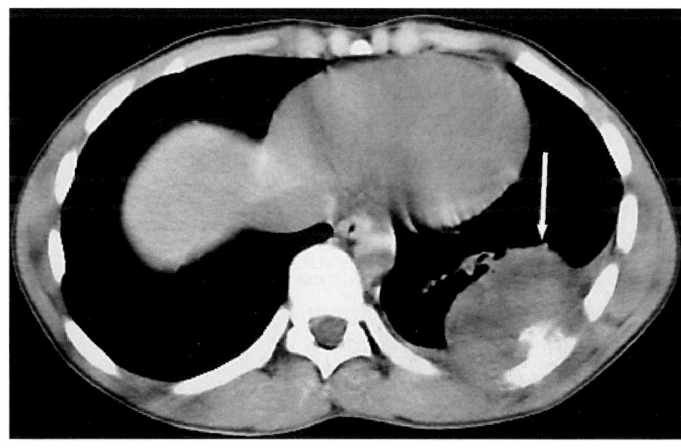

Fig. 41. Conventional Ewing's sarcoma. Radiological features. CT of the chest with the patient in a supine position. There is destruction of the dorsal part of a left-sided rib with a large soft tissue component bulging into the pleural cavity (arrow).

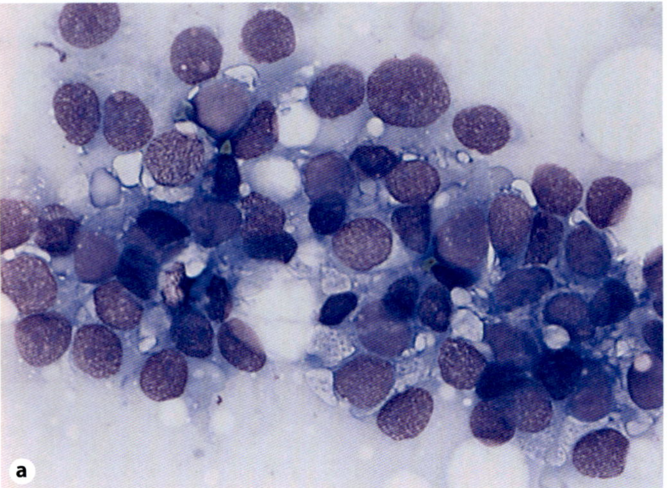

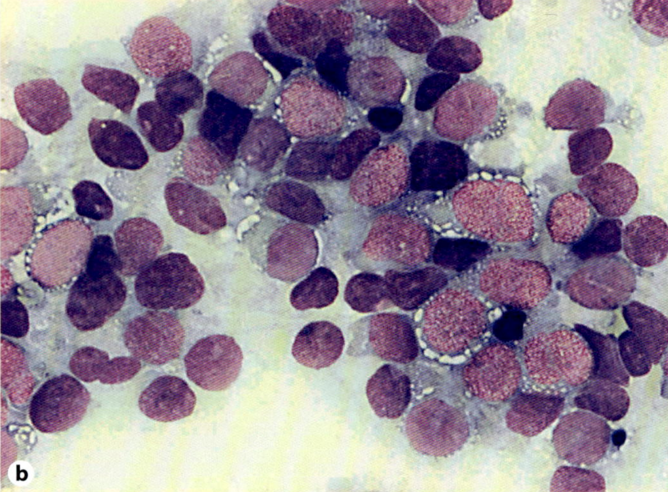

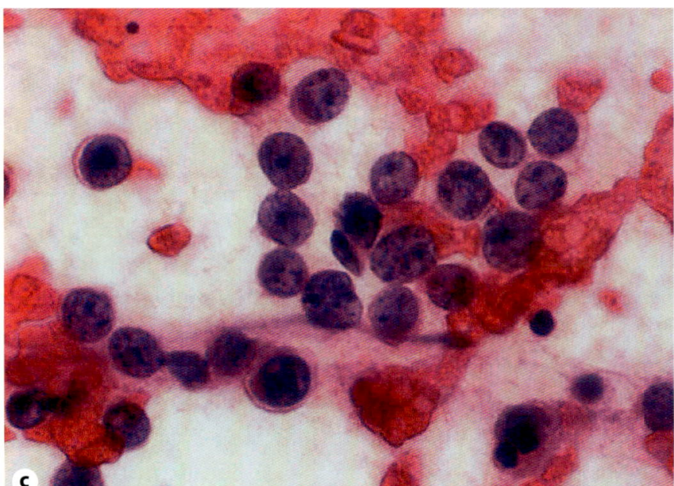

Fig. 42. Conventional Ewing's sarcoma. **a**, **b** Clusters of cohesive tumour cells. Large light cells with vacuolated or clear cytoplasm mixed with small dark cells with sparse cytoplasm and dark irregular nuclei. MGG, medium magnification. **c** The 2 cell types are less evident in wet-fixed smears. The nuclear features, however, are better illustrated: finely granular chromatin, small nucleoli. HE, medium magnification.

component is usually prominent with growth surrounding the entire bone.

The changes in the bone are very well demonstrated by CT. CT is, however, less suitable for investigation of the soft tissues and bone marrow. MRI is mandatory for the evaluation of soft tissue, cortical bone and bone marrow involvement. The tumour enhances with gadolinium-containing contrast media. When EFT appears as a soft tissue mass it cannot radiologically be distinguished from any other type of soft tissue sarcoma.

Histopathology

Conventional Ewing's sarcoma is composed of rather uniform small cells seen either in sheets of cells in a fibrovascular stroma or forming a lobulated pattern. The cellular morphology has been thoroughly described by Angerwall and Enzinger [60] who emphasized the double cell population, which are large, cytoplasm-rich cells with abundant cytoplasm and nuclei with finely granular chromatin and insignificant nucleoli (principal cells are large light cells) and another population of smaller cells with sparse cytoplasm and irregular, dark nuclei (small dark cells). The principal cells contain more or less abundant cytoplasmic glycogen. Homer-Wright-like rosettes are rarely present. Mitoses are usually infrequent. Atypical Ewing's sarcoma and PNET display more marked anisokaryosis with different grades of nuclear atypia, prominent nucleoli and less cytoplasmic glycogen. Spindled cells with cytoplasmic extensions as well as rhabdomyoblast-like cells and cells with rhabdoid morphology may be observed. Mitoses are more frequently found compared to conventional Ewing's sarcoma and a double cell population is often not evident. Rosettes are easily found, especially in PNET.

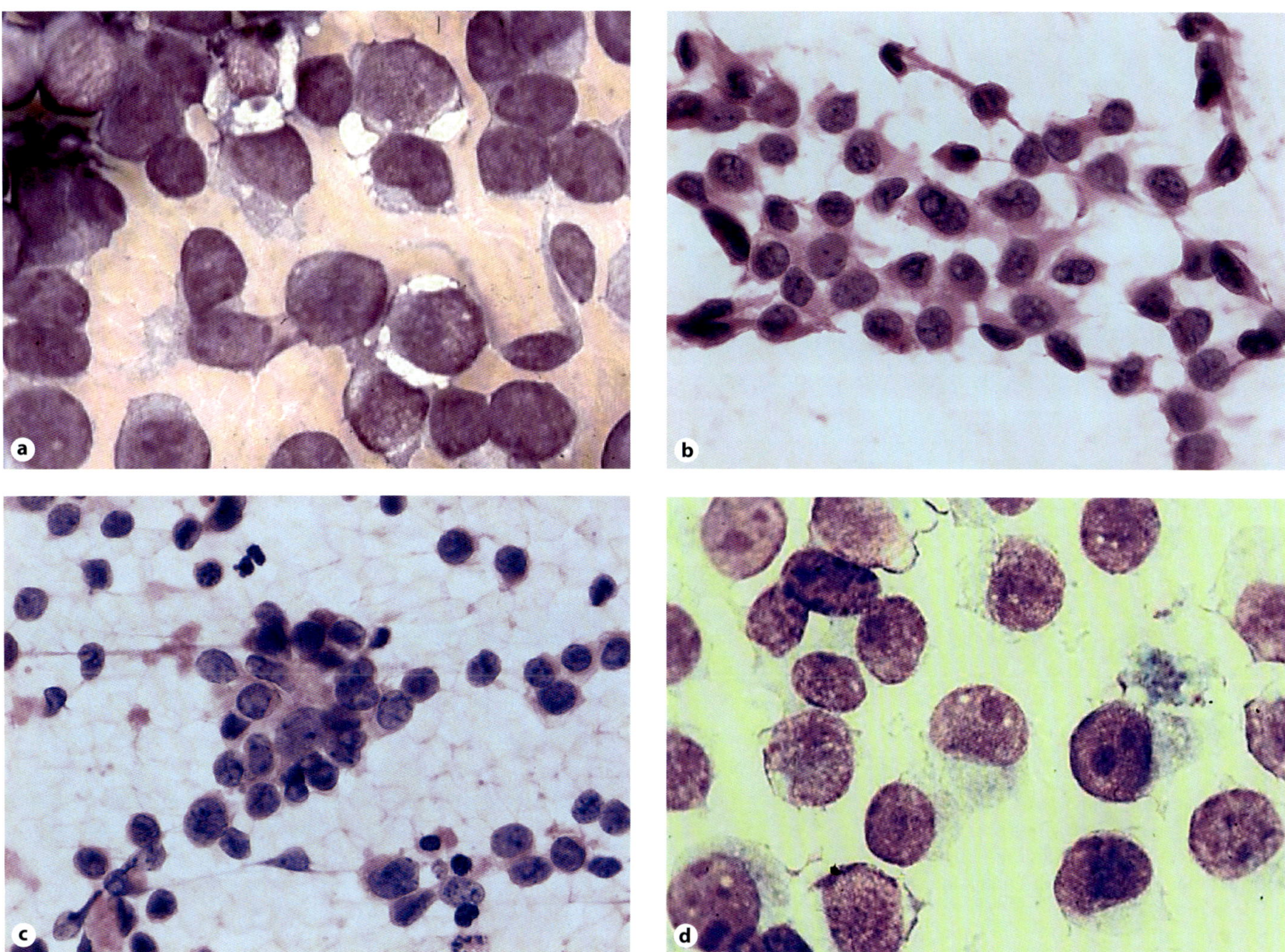

Fig. 43. Atypical Ewing's sarcoma and PNET. **a** The distinction between the 2 cell types is less evident. There are scattered cells with vacuolated cytoplasm. Moderate cellular and nuclear atypia. MGG, high magnification. **b** Tumour cells with long cytoplasmic processes may be part of the cytological spectrum. HE, medium magnification. **c** Rosettes composed of atypical cells are often present. HE, low magnification. **d** The cellular pleomorphism may be marked with prominent nucleoli. Rhabdomyoblast-like cells may be part of the cellular spectrum. MGG, high magnification.

Cytological Features of Classical Ewing's Sarcoma

See figure 42. Frequently there are cellular aspirates. Dispersed cells are admixed with clusters or groups of loosely cohesive cells. Fragile cells are seen, striped nuclei are present and background matrix is cytoplasmic. There are 2 cell types: (1) large cells with abundant, 'thin' cytoplasm with clear spaces or vacuoles and rounded nuclei with finely chromatin texture and small nucleoli, and (2) small dark cells with hyperchromatic nuclei and scanty cytoplasm. There is cytoplasmic glycogen in the large cells. Occasionally rosette-like structures are seen.

Cytological Features of Atypical Ewing's Sarcoma and PNET

See figure 43. The 2 cell types outlined above are less evident. There is a variable degree of cellular pleomorphism (more marked in PNET) including anisokaryosis, hyperchromasia and prominent nucleoli. Spindle-shaped cells with cytoplasmic extensions are present. Rhabdomyoblast-like tumour cells and tumour cells with rhabdoid morphology may be present. In PNET, mitoses and rosette-like structures are not uncommon.

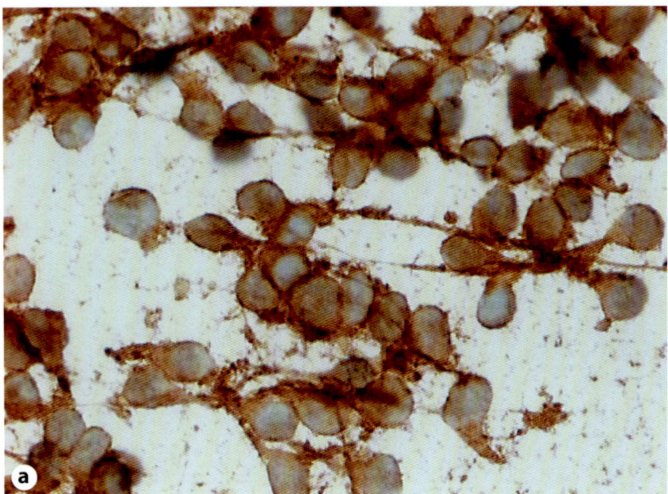

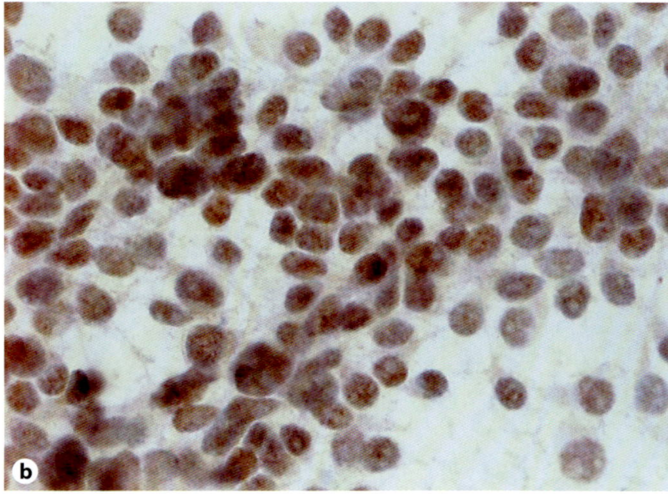

Fig. 44. a The tumour cells are strongly positive for CD99. Cytospin preparation, immunoperoxidase, medium magnification. **b** The tumour cell nuclei are strongly positive for Fli-1. Cytospin preparation, immunoperoxidase, medium magnification.

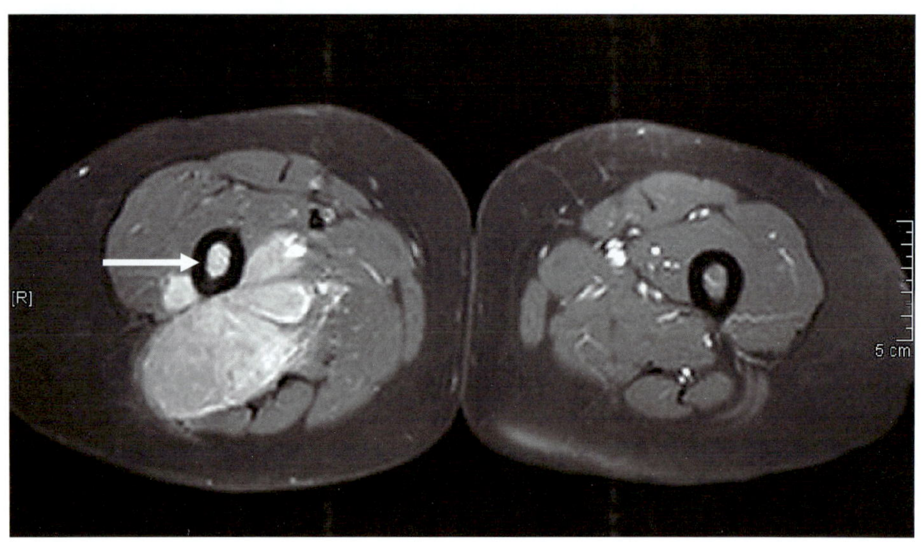

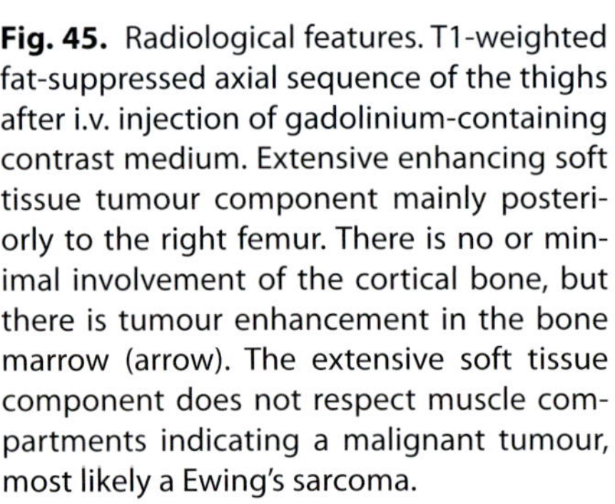

Fig. 45. Radiological features. T1-weighted fat-suppressed axial sequence of the thighs after i.v. injection of gadolinium-containing contrast medium. Extensive enhancing soft tissue tumour component mainly posteriorly to the right femur. There is no or minimal involvement of the cortical bone, but there is tumour enhancement in the bone marrow (arrow). The extensive soft tissue component does not respect muscle compartments indicating a malignant tumour, most likely a Ewing's sarcoma.

Differential Diagnosis

The differential diagnoses are: neuroblastoma; estesioneuroblastoma; alveolar rhabdomyosarcoma; non-Hodgkin lymphoma (precursor lymphoma); desmoplastic small round cell tumour; poorly differentiated Ewing's sarcoma-like synovial sarcoma; small-cell osteosarcoma, and mesenchymal chondrosarcoma.

Comments

The cytological diagnostic criteria of conventional Ewing's sarcoma and PNET have been reported in several publications [15, 61–67]. In our opinion, a correct diagnosis of classical Ewing's sarcoma is possible on routine stained, adequate and technically satisfactory smears provided that air-dried as well as wet-fixed material is examined. The double cell population is characteristic and remarkably repetitive from case to case. The cytoplasmic features of the large cells (cytoplasmic abundance, vacuoles, clear spaces) are best visualized in MGG or DiffQuick while the nuclear characteristics are better seen in HE or Pap. When only wet-fixed material is available classical Ewing's sarcoma may be difficult to distinguish from poorly differentiated synovial sarcoma with Ewing's sarcoma-like cells.

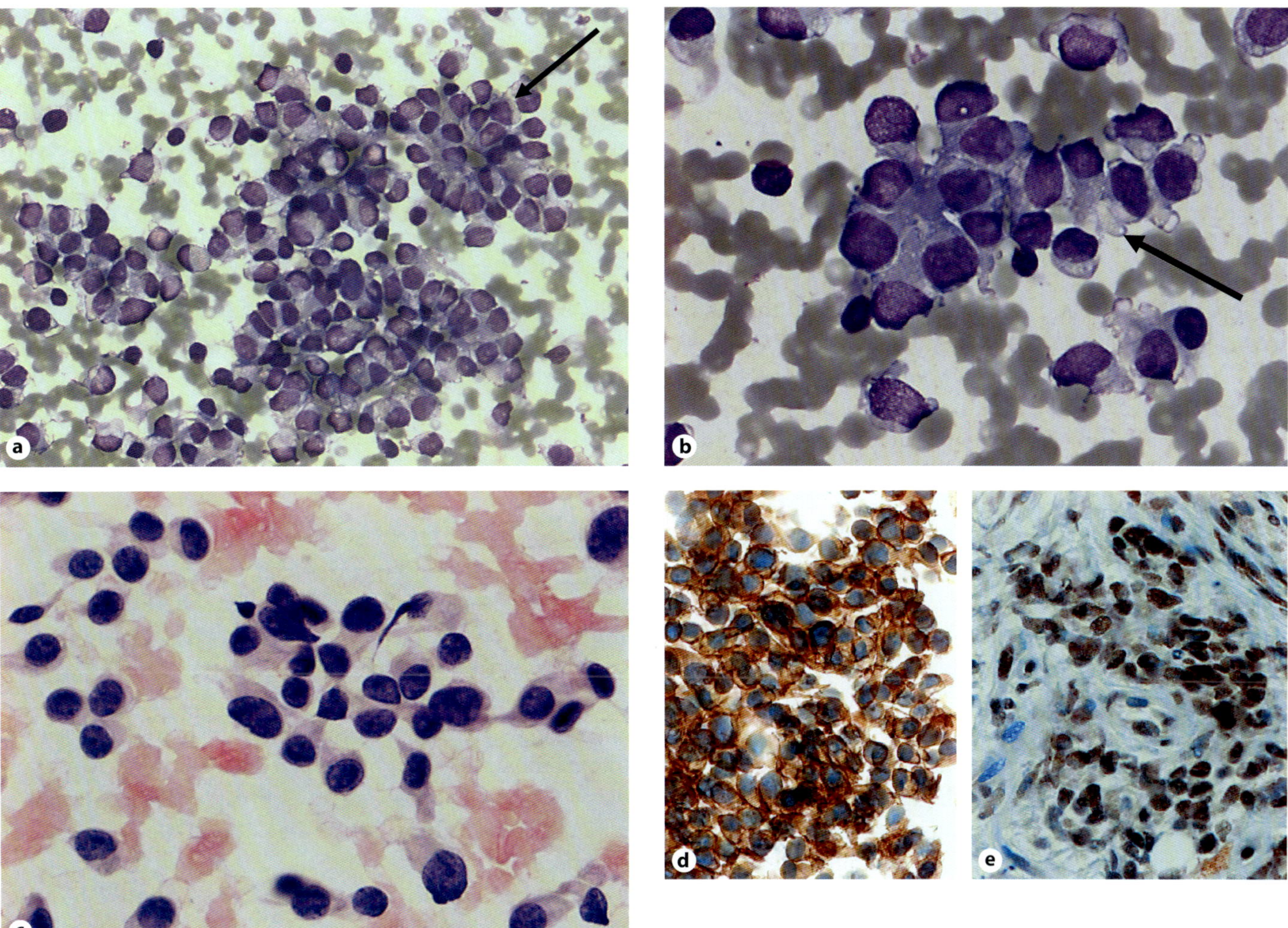

Fig. 46. **a** A cohesive cluster of small tumour cells. A rosette-like structure is present in the upper right corner (arrow). MGG, low magnification. **b** The tumour cells have rather abundant cytoplasm with clear spaces (arrow) and eccentric nuclei. MGG, high magnification. **c** The wet-fixed smear shows moderately atypical, rounded or irregular nuclei with coarse chromatin. HE, high magnification. **d** The tumour cells are strongly positive for CD99. Cell block preparation, immunoperoxidase, low magnification. **e** The tumour cell nuclei are strongly positive for Fli-1. Cell block preparation, immunoperoxidase, low magnification.

In atypical Ewing's sarcoma and PNET, the pleomorphism and cellular and nuclear atypia make it difficult to give a definitive, correct diagnosis of EFT although this diagnosis might be strongly suspected. The clinical setting decides to some extent which of the possible differential diagnoses is the most relevant in a given case. For example, neuroblastoma in children below the age of 5, estesioneuroblastoma in nasopharyngeal tumours, desmoplastic small-round-cell tumour in abdominal lesions. Frequently, skeletal EFT presents with a soft tissue extension, which can be misinterpreted as a true soft tissue tumour prior to radiological investigation. The distinction between small-cell osteosarcoma and EFT is difficult, and the presence of osteoid in the smears is of help in the differential diagnosis. Mesenchymal chondrosarcoma is a differential diagnostic problem in those cases where the small-cell population predominates and fragments of hyaline cartilage are difficult to find.

Although classical Ewing's sarcoma can be reliably diagnosed on routine stained smears, ancillary methods are strongly recommended to supplement the routine cytological evaluation of tumours suggestive of EFT. CD99 and FLI-1 are considered highly sensitive (fig. 44), but unfortunately non-specific, antibodies in the diagnosis of EFT [59, 60]. CD99 and FLI-1 must be used together with a panel of other antibodies, especially when alveolar rhabdomyosarcoma, precursor lymphoma, abdominal small-round-cell tumour and poorly differentiated synovial sarcoma are part of the differential diagnostic spectrum [68]. Demonstration of the characteristic chromosomal aberration is the gold standard for diagnosing EFT according to many investigators. Ordinary karyotyping, RT-PCR and fluorescence in situ hybridization (FISH) have all been tested on FNA material. Best results have been achieved with RT-PCR and FISH. In our own experience RT-PCR and FISH are most suitable for FNA samples. When aspirated material is sufficient for RT-PCR and FISH, respectively resulting in the EWS/FLI-1 transcript and split EWS signal, the diagnosis is reliably established. In cases of abdominal small-round-cell tumour versus EFT, FISH is less reliable as the genotype of the abdominal small cell tumour, t(11;22)(p13;q12), also involves the EWS gene (the EWS/WT-1 transcript).

Case Report 4

The patient was a middle-aged female with a 1-year history of a tumour in the right thigh. Clinical examination revealed a deep-seated large (10 × 10 × 5 cm) palpable soft-tissue tumour.

Radiological examination was a T1-weighted fat-suppressed axial sequence of the thighs after i.v. injection of gadolinium-containing contrast medium (fig. 45). It showed an extensive enhancing soft tissue component of a tumour located mainly dorsal to the right femur. There was no or minimally involvement of the cortical bone, but there was tumour enhancement in the bone marrow (arrow in the figure).The extensive soft tissue component did not respect muscle compartments, indicating a malignant tumour, most likely Ewing's sarcoma.

FNA was performed by the cytopathologist.

Figure 46a (MGG, low magnification) shows a cohesive cluster of small tumour cells. A rosette-like structure is present in the upper right corner (arrow). Figure 46b (MGG, high magnification) shows the tumour cells have rather abundant cytoplasm with clear spaces (arrow) and eccentric irregular nuclei. In figure 46c (HE, high magnification) moderately atypical, rounded or irregular nuclei with coarse chromatin are depicted in the wet-fixed smear. In figure 46d (cell-block preparation, immunoperoxidase) the tumour cells are strongly positive for CD99. In figure 46e (cell-block preparation, immunoperoxidase) the tumour cell nuclei are strongly positive for Fli-1.

The cytological diagnosis was EFT (atypical Ewing's sarcoma). A core needle biopsy was performed showing the same immunophenotype.

Comments

Clinically this tumour presented itself as a soft-tissue tumour but the radiological investigation clearly demonstrated a tumour in the femoral bone with extensive soft tissue involvement, which is not uncommon in EFT.

The cytoplasmic clear spaces in the tumour cells, the presence of rosette-like structures, and the absence of osteoid-like intercellular matrix favoured an EFT more than other diagnostic alternatives, such as small-cell osteosarcoma, primary non-Hodgkin lymphoma or metastasis of alveolar rhabdomyosarcoma.

The unequivocal expression of CD99 and Fli-1 in the tumour cells strongly favoured an EFT. The evident although moderate cellular and nuclear atypia and the absence of a typical double cell population (large light and small dark cells) indicated an atypical Ewing's sarcoma or PNET rather than a classical Ewing's sarcoma.

Chapter 8

Cytological Features of Bone Tumours in FNA Smears IV: Notochordal Tumours

Chordoma

Chordoma, which arises from remnants of the notochord, is a rare bone tumour that accounts for up to 4% of the primary bone sarcomas. Chordoma is most common in the sixth and seventh decades and is very rare under the age of 30. Chordoma arises in the axial spine, sacrum is the most common site, followed by the spheno-occipital area, cervical spine and thoraco-lumbar spine.

Radiology

See figure 47. Chordomas are often difficult to diagnose by conventional radiology, due to the fact that bowel gas and content obscure the outlining of the sacrum. Large chordomas may be overlooked. CT and MRI are the methods of choice to diagnose and to outline these tumours. In the sacrum the tumour destroys the cortex of the anterior and posterior faces, often with a large soft tissue component. Calcifications are commonly found. When chordomas occur in a vertebra, the radiological findings are those of bone destruction. Whichever the site, there is often growth into the spinal canal.

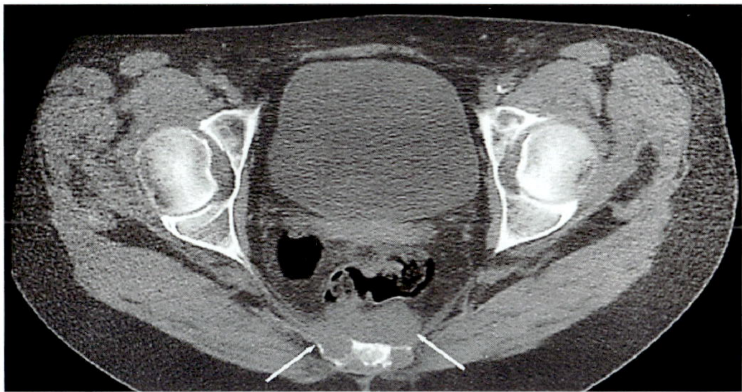

Fig. 47. Chordoma. Radiological features. Axial CT of the pelvis. There is a tumour around the tip of the sacrum with relatively mild destruction of bone in this section. The soft tissue component is indicated by arrows.

Histopathology

See figure 48. Chordomas have a lobulated growth pattern, the tumour lobules are separated by fibrous bands. An abundant myxoid matrix is always present. The tumour cells are arranged in sheets or cords or seen as single elements floating in the background matrix. Typical tumour cells are large with abundant (multi)vacuolated cytoplasm and rounded or ovoid nuclei (physaliferous cells). The physaliferous cells are admixed with smaller, epithelioid-like cells and spindly cells. Cellular atypia is usually not prominent although multinucleated tumour giant cells and cells with hyperchromasia and prominent nucleoli may be present.

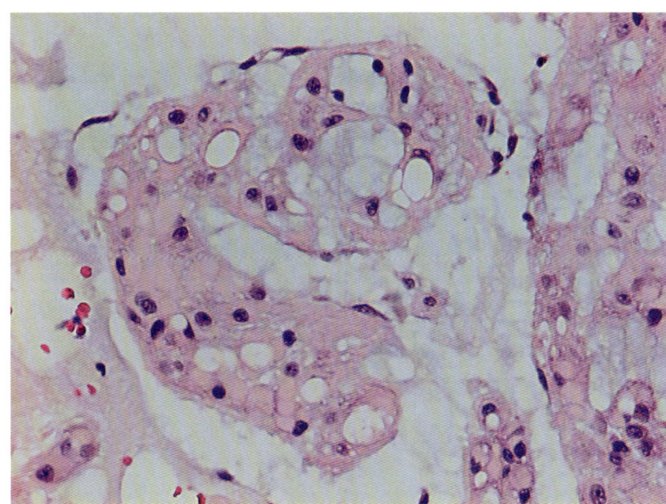

Fig. 48. Chordoma. Histology. Groups and cords of large cells with abundant cytoplasm and moderately atypical nuclei are embedded in a faintly stained myxoid back-ground matrix. (HE Medium magnification.)

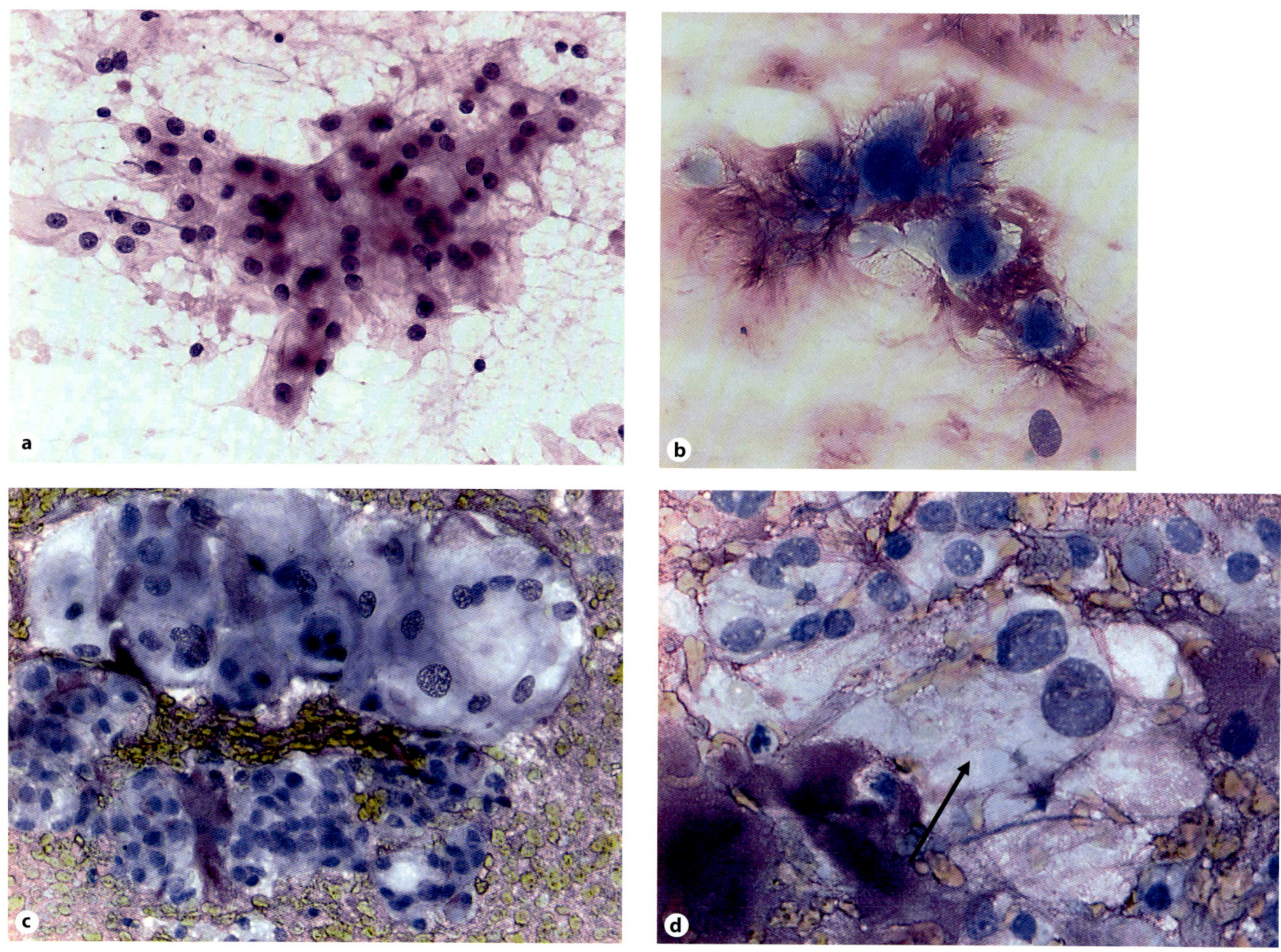

Fig. 49. a A cluster of tumour cells embedded in a fibrillar myxoid matrix. HE, low magnification. **b** The fibrillar matrix encircles single tumour cells. MGG, medium magnification. **c, d** The tumour cells are large with abundant cytoplasm. Typical physaliferous cells are present in **d** (arrow). MGG, high magnification.

Immunohistochemically chordomas stain with S-100 protein, low molecular cytokeratins (CK8 and 18) and EMA.

Cytological Features

See figure 49. There is abundant myxoid background matrix, characteristically encircling tumour cell groups and single tumour cells. Large, cytoplasm-rich cells with (multi)vacuolated cytoplasm (physaliferous cells) are evident. There are strands, groups or clusters of medium-sized rounded, epithelial-like cells, at times binucleated. Spindle cells are infrequent. Nuclei are rounded or ovoid, there is moderate anisokaryosis, bland chromatin and nucleoli are small. Pleomorphic, atypical tumour cells with large nucleoli are seen, as well as multinucleated tumour giant cells in some tumours.

Differential Diagnosis

The differential diagnoses are chondrosarcoma, clear cell- or mucin-producing adenocarcinoma, and myxopapillary ependymoma.

Comments

Although chordoma is a rare primary bone sarcoma, 4 relatively large series of chordomas investigated by FNA have been published [15, 69–72]. The characteristic features are the abundant, myxoid, often fibrillar background substance, which like a network encircles groups of cells and/or single tumour cells and the presence of the physaliferous cells with their abundant 'bubbly' cytoplasm and rounded nuclei with inconspicuous nucleoli. Clusters or groups of medium-sized, rounded, epithelial-like cells with rounded or ovoid

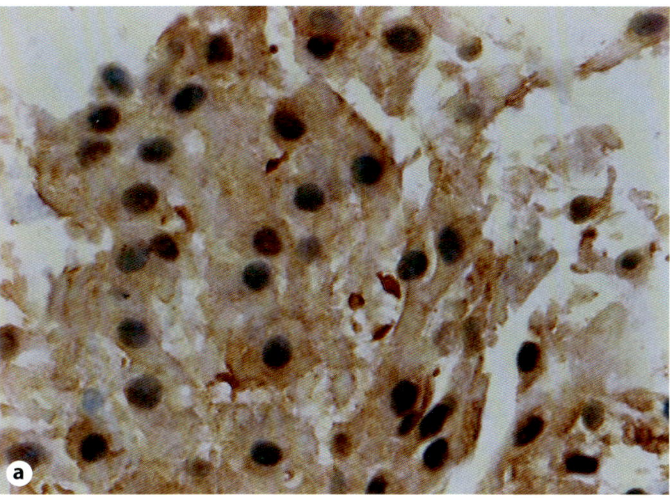

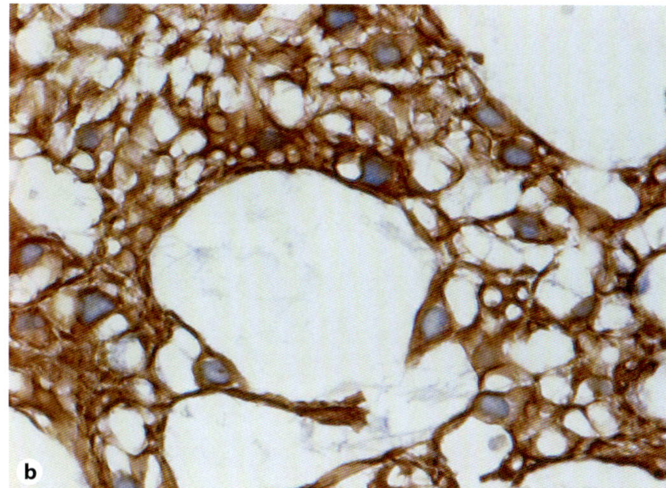

Fig. 50. Tumour cells are positive for S-100 protein (**a**) and cytokeratin (**b**; MNF). Cell block preparation, immunoperoxidase, low magnification.

nuclei are also present. These cells may be vacuolated with eccentric, at times scalloped nuclei, resembling lipoblasts or signet-ring cells in adenocarcinoma. The myxoid matrix is intensely red-blue or violet in MGG and DiffQuick, pale pink in HE and pale green-grey in Pap. In wet-fixed smears the background matrix is much less obvious than in air-dried smears and this feature, together with the presence of epithelioid-like cells, sometimes vacuolated with eccentric nuclei, might lead to an incorrect diagnosis of metastastic adenocarcinoma. Typical physaliferous cells are not seen in chondrosarcoma, nor the fibrillar matrix encircling individual tumour cells. Saccrococcygeal myxopapillary ependymoma is another, albeit very rare, differential diagnosis. In the few cases of FNAC reported of this rare tumour, central mucin cores surrounded by cuboidal or columnar cells in a rosette-like pattern was a typical finding, and physaliphorus cells were not present [73–75].

Chordomas in the cervical spine may present as eccentric (not midline) tumours and, in the absence of radiographic findings, may be interpreted as soft tissue myxoid sarcomas, especially in cases with pleomorphic atypical tumour cells or multinucleated giant tumour cells.

Immunocytochemistry is of great help in the differential diagnosis from chondrosarcoma.

Chordomas typically express S-100 protein together with EMA and/or low molecular weight keratin (fig. 50). As some carcinomas may express S-100 protein, distinction from metastatic adenocarcinoma can be problematic. Chordoma does not express carcinoembryonic antigen, which helps to exclude metastatic gastrointestinal carcinoma.

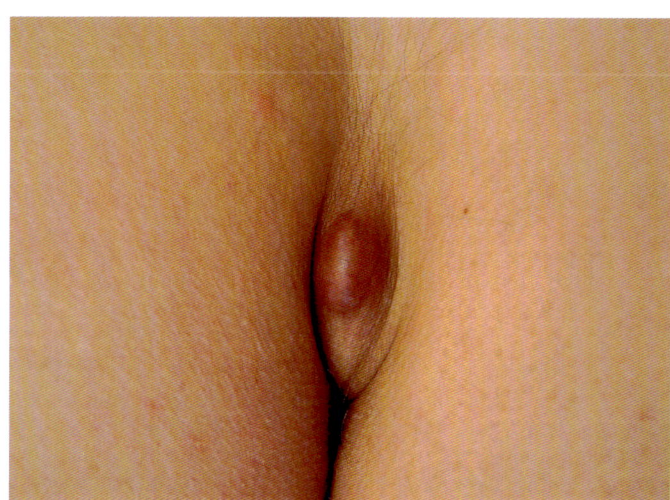

Fig. 51. The patient presented with a soft tissue tumour in the crena ani.

Case Report 5

The patient was a middle-aged male with low back pain. A palpable soft tissue tumour was found in the crena ani on clinical investigation (fig. 51).

FNA was performed by the cytopathologist.

Figure 52a, b (MGG, high manification) shows large tumour cells with abundant cytoplasm and rounded nuclei embedded in a myxoid background matrix. The abundant cytoplasm is vacuolated. Note the thin matrix threads encircling the tumour cells. In figure 52c (HE, high magnification)

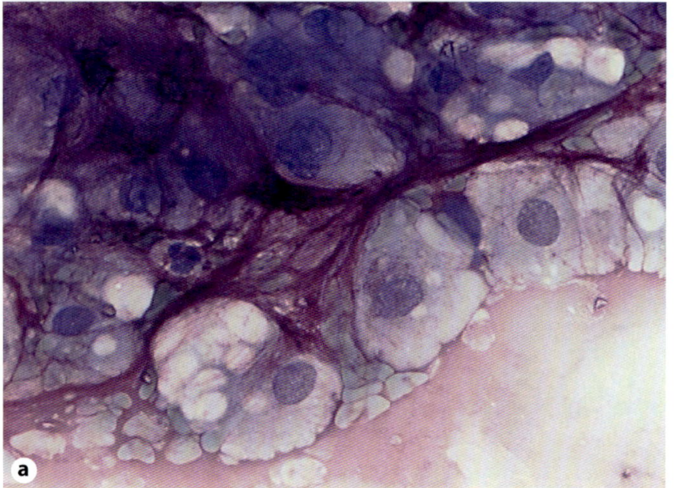

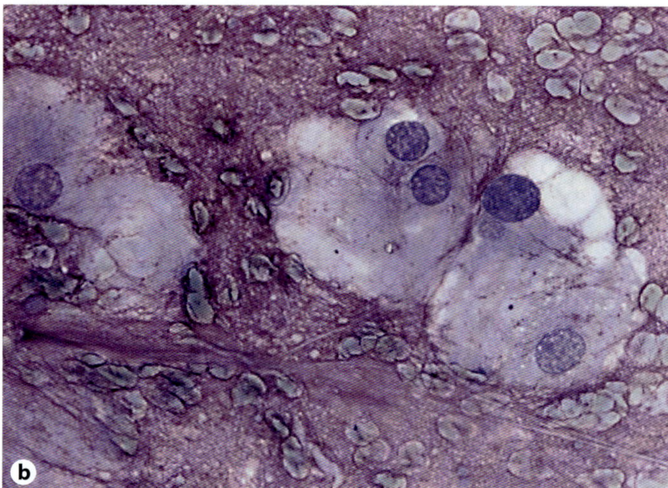

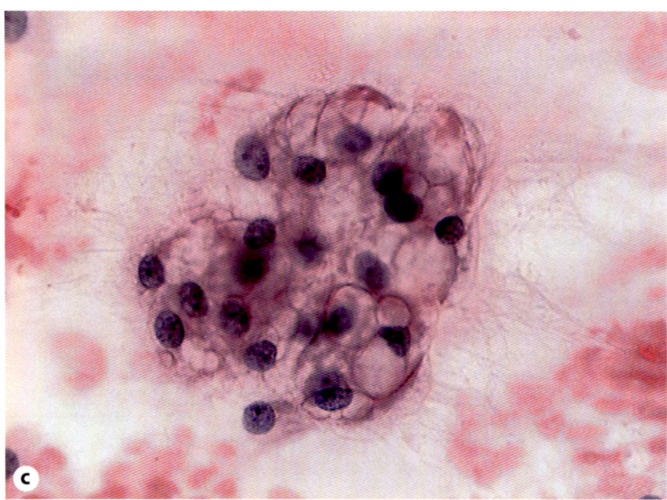

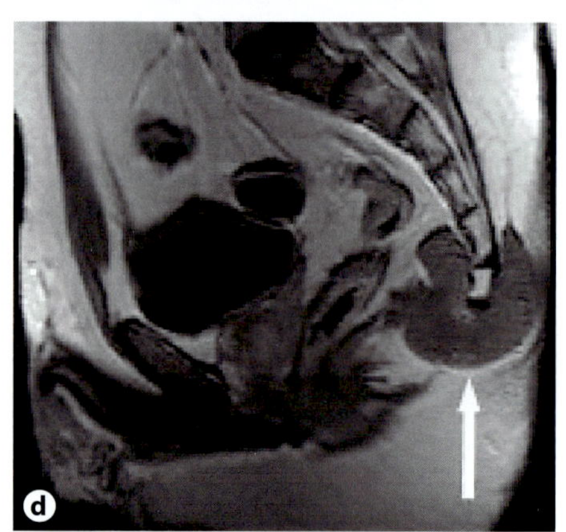

Fig. 52. a, **b**. Large tumour cells with abundant cytoplasm and rounded nuclei embedded in a myxoid background matrix. The abundant cytoplasm is vacuolated. Note thin matrix threads encircling the tumour cells. MGG, high magnification. **c** The tumour cells have rather uniform nuclei with small nucleoli. The vacuolated cytoplasm is well visible in the wet-fixed smear but the abundant myxoid back-ground matrix is almost not visible in HE. HE, high magnification. **d**. Subsequent sagittal MRI of the tumour in a T1-weighted sequence. A lesion surrounding the tip of the sacrum infiltrating in the soft tissues dorsal to the sacrum is seen (arrow). In this sequence the tumour is dark. The radiological features are compatible with a chordoma.

the tumour cells have rather uniform nuclei with small nucleoli. The vacuolated cytoplasm is easily visible in the wet-fixed smear but the abundant myxoid background matrix is almost not visible in HE.

Although the tumour presented as a soft tissue tumour, the cellular features combined with the abundant myxoid matrix suggested a chordoma.

Figure 52d shows a subsequent axial MRI of the tumour in a T1-weighted sequence. A lesion surrounding the tip of the sacrum infiltrating in the soft tissues dorsal to the sacrum is seen (arrow). In this sequence the tumour is dark. The radiological features are compatible with a chordoma.

The cytological diagnosis was sacral chordoma.

Comments

Chordomas might, according to our experience, present themselves as true soft tissue tumours, especially in the cervical spine, and are then often needled without previous radiological investigation. In those instances, the most important differential diagnoses are the myxoid soft-tissue sarcomas. The HE-stained smear in figure 52c demonstrates that chordoma cells might look like vacuolated carcinoma cells and that the typical myxoid chordoma matrix is almost invisible in wet-fixed smears.

Chapter 9

Cytological Features of Bone Tumours in FNA Smears V: Giant-Cell Lesions

Conventional Giant-Cell Tumour

Giant-cell tumour is an infrequent bone tumour, comprising approximately 5% primary bone tumours. Most patients are 20–60 years of age, with the peak between 20 and 40 years. The conventional giant cell tumour is usually an epiphyseal lesion, most often appearing in the distal part of the femur, proximal part of the tibia and in the distal part of the radius. It is very rare in the spine but not uncommon in the sacrum. Although giant cell tumours are benign tumours, they may occasionally give rise to tumour deposits in the lungs.

Radiology

See figure 53. Giant-cell tumours typically grow eccentrically, usually close to the subchondral bone and may penetrate into the adjacent joint. They are lytic, the cortical outline is often thin and may seem destroyed, but the tumour is almost always outlined and defined by the periosteum. Depending on the size and the thickness of the cortex there is an increased risk for fractures.

Histopathology

The typical pattern is that of a tumour with a vascular stroma and ovoid, rounded or spindle-shaped mononuclear cells interspersed with multinucleated giant cells which may contain up to 50 nuclei. The stromal and giant-cell nuclei are

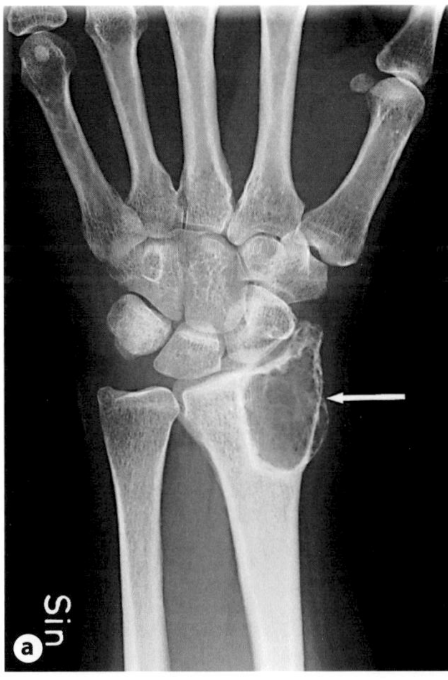

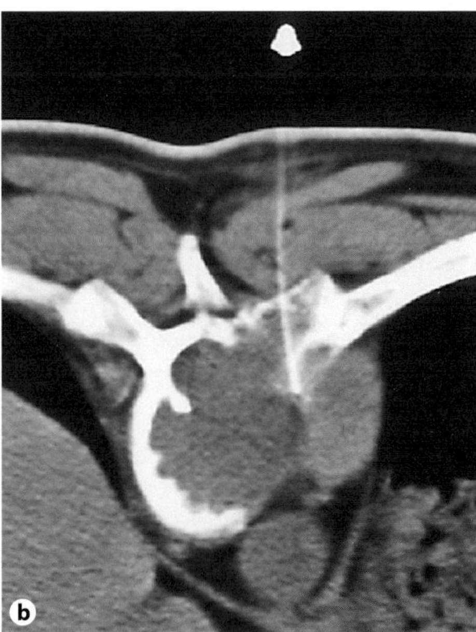

Fig. 53. a, b Giant cell tumour. Radiological features. **a** PA radiograph of the left wrist. There is a lytic lesion located eccentrically at the distal end of radius, involving the epiphysis and the metaphysis. The lesion is also located subchondrally to the wrist joint and is well demarcated with a thin sclerotic rim. **b** CT of the thoracic spine with the patient in prone position. There is an extensive destruction of the ninth vertebral body, including the right pedicle and the right cortex of the vertebral body. There is also a right-sided soft tissue component. Note the FNA needle inserted in the tumour.

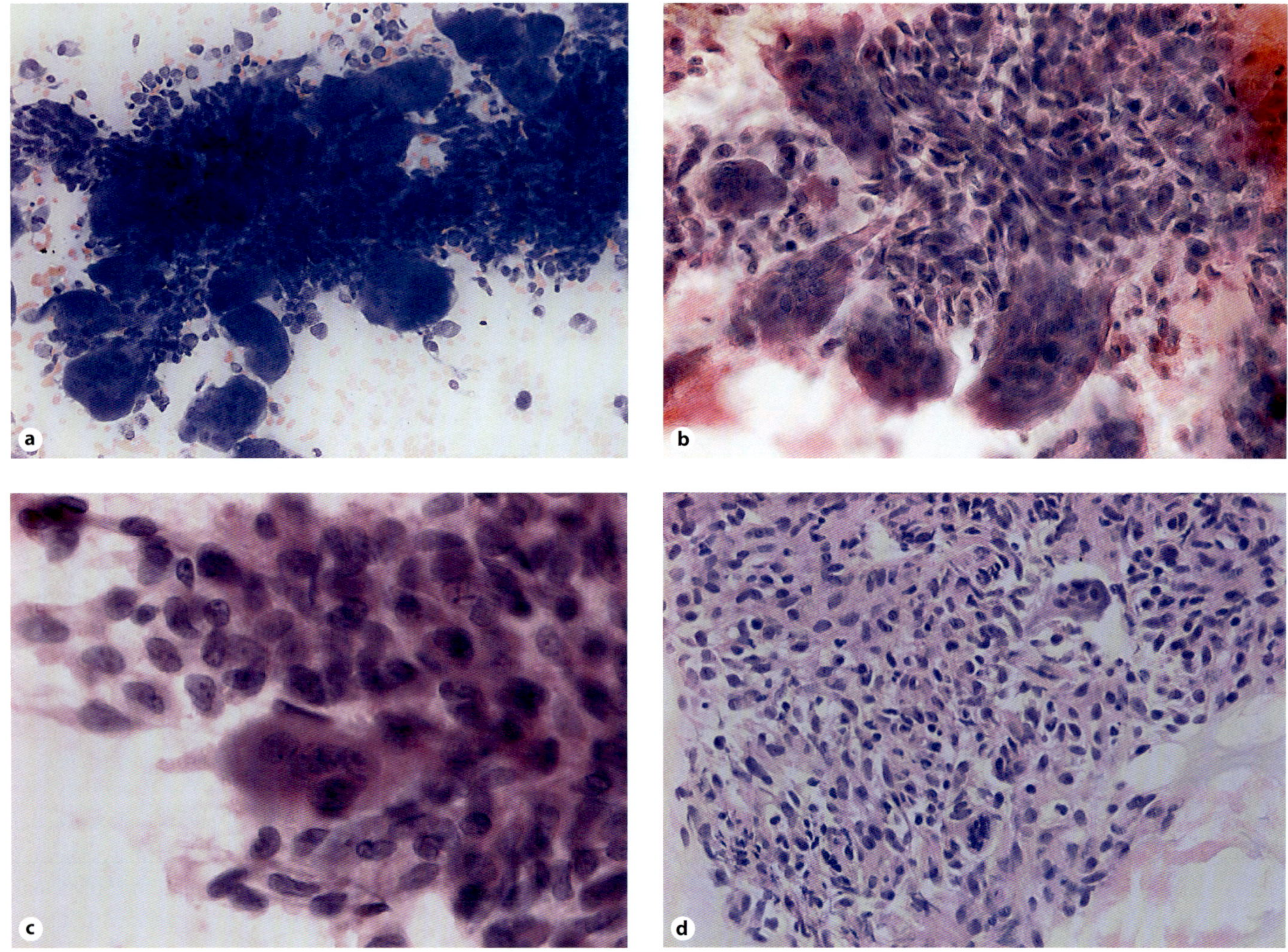

Fig. 54. Cohesive cell clusters bordered by multiple multinucleated giant cells. **a** MGG, low magnification. **b** HE, low magnification. **c** The mononuclear cells are rounded, ovoid or spindly with slightly pleomorphic nuclei. HE, medium magnification. **d** Cell block preparation from the same case. The aspirated material corresponds well with the mini-biopsy. HE, low magnification.

similar, being rounded or ovoid with finely granular chromatin and prominent nucleoli. Mitoses are not uncommon in the stromal cells, but atypical mitoses should not be present. The tumour does not produce bone or cartilaginous matrix. This typical histological pattern is often modified by haemorrhage, necrosis or reactive fibrous tissue. Aneurysmal bone cyst like areas may be present.

Cytological Features

See figure 54. There is often abundant yield, with a mixture of cohesive cell clusters and single cells. The double cell population contains mononuclear spindly, rounded or ovoid cells and multinucleated osteoclast-like giant cells. There are slightly pleomorphic nuclei with finely granular chromatin and prominent nucleoli. In typical FNA samples, giant cells are attached to the periphery of clustered mononuclear cells.

Differential Diagnosis

The differential diagnoses are: other benign bone lesions/tumours harbouring osteoclast-like giant cells such as aneurysmal bone cyst, brown tumour of hyperparathyroidism, reparative giant-cell granuloma, osteoblastoma, and giant-cell-rich osteosarcoma.

Comments

Due to their expansive and destructive growth with thinning of the cortical bone, giant-cell tumours are most often easy to needle and the material is abundant. The cytological features of conventional giant-cell tumour as described in 3 series of a total of 38 cases are in accord [15, 76, 77] Although it has been emphasized that clusters of mononuclear cells bordered by giant cells at the periphery is a characteristic cytological feature [77], in our experience this pattern is also present in smears from brown tumours of hyperparathyroidism.

From the clinical point of view, the most important pitfall is giant-cell-rich osteosarcoma. When the material is abundant, the marked atypia of the tumour cells of giant-cell-rich osteosarcoma prevents a false benign diagnosis, but in smears with numerous giant cells and few mononuclear cells it is wise not to make a definitive diagnosis of giant-cell tumour even if suggested by radiological imaging. With regard to the differential diagnosis of other benign tumours/lesions with numerous giant cells, full knowledge of clinical and radiographic data is essential for a correct type-specific diagnosis.

Aneurysmal Bone Cyst

Primary aneurysmal bone cyst is a multilocular, benign but locally destructive lesion. Aneurysmal bone cyst is less common than conventional giant-cell tumour and the majority of cases occur in patients up to 30 years of age with the highest incidence in the second decade. Any bone can be affected but more than 60% arise in the vertebral column, the craniofascial bones and the long tubular bones.

Secondary aneurysmal bone cyst is an aneurysmal bone cyst which is found together with another tumour/lesion such as giant-cell tumour, spinal osteoblastoma, chondroblastoma and chondromyxoid fibroma.

Radiology
See figure 55. Aneurysmal bone cysts are most often located in the metaphyses of the long bones. In the spine any level, including the sacrum, may be involved but they mainly affect the posterior elements of the vertebrae. The tumour is eccentrically located, lytic and surrounded by a rim of sclerosis. The cortical surface of the affected bone is expanded and ballooned. The cortical definition may be lost and with the extension into the adjacent soft tissue it may appear as a malignant tumour. With CT and MRI, characteristic localized fluid levels may be seen within the cystic spaces. The cystic cavities may appear on plain radiography as thin sclerotic trabeculae. Radiologically, the lesion can be confused with a giant-cell tumour but the localization is different in the long bones.

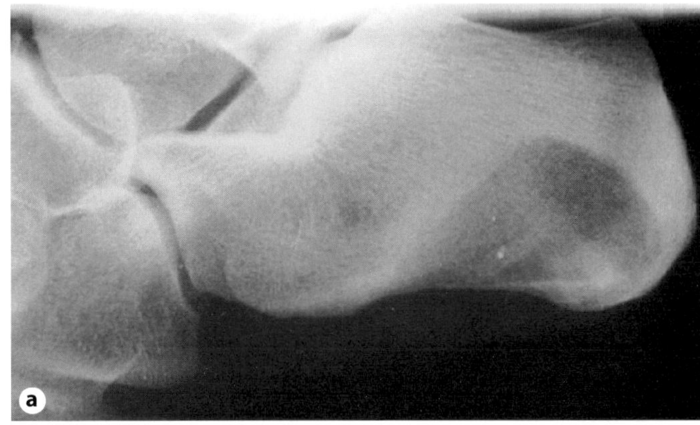

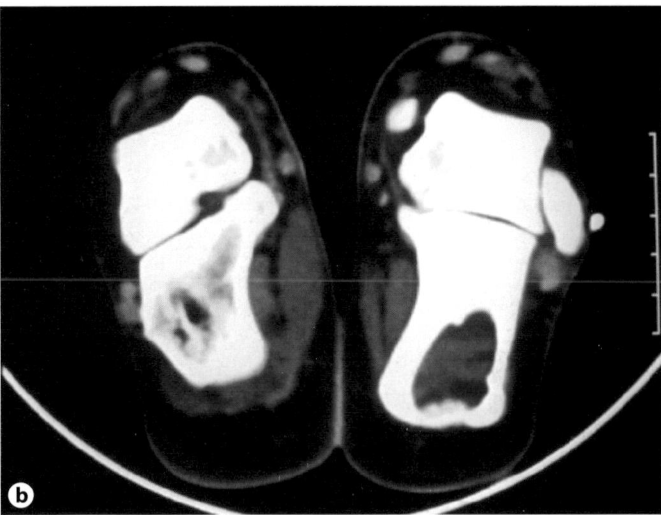

Fig. 55. Aneurysmal bone cyst. Radiological features. **a** Radiograph of the left calcaneus in lateral projection. There is a well demarcated lytic lesion without sclerotic margins. **b** Axial CT of the heel. The lytic lesion contains compartments with separate fluid levels (arrow), a characteristic CT or MRI finding of aneurysmal bone cyst.

Histopathology
See figure 56. Fragments of fibrous septa and solid tissue areas are seen on a hemorrhagic background. Both septae and solid areas are composed of vascular fibrous tissue with multinucleated giant cells and inflammatory cells. Focal reactive bone formation is common, including reactive osteoid and reactive osteoblasts.

Cytological Features
See figure 57. Aspirates are haemorrhagic aspirates, with variable numbers of multinucleated giant cells and variable presence of spindle cells in clusters. Histiocytes and inflammatory cells are seen.

Differential Diagnoses
The differential diagnoses are: conventional giant-cell tumour; solitary bone cyst; giant-cell reparative granuloma, and brown tumour of hyperparathyroidism.

Comments
The cytological features of primary aneurysmal bone cyst have been recorded in single cases [78]. In our experience, most aneurysmal bone cysts are diagnosed as benign tumours with osteoclast-like giant cells or as solitary bone cysts. A specific diagnosis depends on radiographic signs.

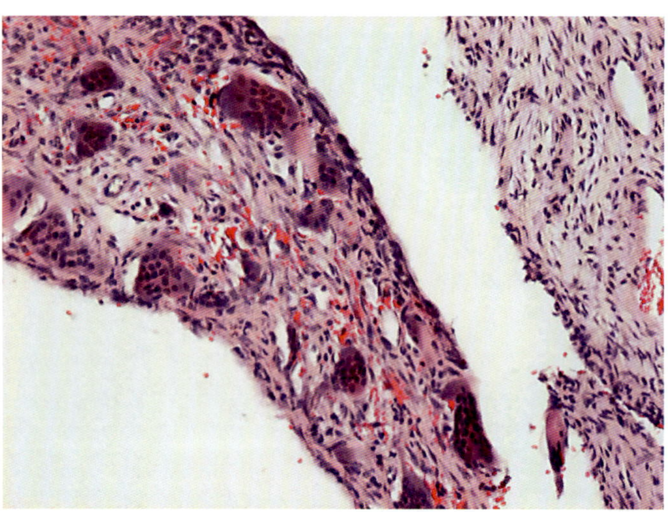

Fig. 56. Histology. Fibrous septa and solid areas composed of vascular fibrous tissue with the presence of multiple osteoclast-like multinucleated giant cells. HE, medium magnification.

Giant-Cell Reparative Granuloma

This is a benign reactive lesion principally occurring in the craniofascial bones and the small tubular bones of the hands and feet. Giant cell reparative granuloma may occur in normal bone or in pre-existing lesions, such as brown tumour of hyperparathyroidism, or secondary to trauma or haemorrhage. Some investigators claim that the so-called solid variant of aneurysmal bone cyst and giant cell-reparative granuloma represents the same reactive process [30]. Most patients are between 10 and 30 years of age.

Radiology
See figure 58. The lesions are lytic and expansile and involve the metaphysis and diaphysis, but can expand to the epiphysis. The overlying cortex is thin, but not destroyed. There are no calcifications. Radiologically, giant cell reparative granuloma may resemble several other entities, including giant cell tumour, aneurysmal bone cyst, brown tumour of hyperparathyroidism and enchondroma.

Histopathology
See figure 59. This lesion is made up of fibrous tissue with spindle shaped (myo)fibroblasts and unevenly distributed multinucleated giant cells, the giant cells are often clustered. Microscopic sequelae of haemorrhage

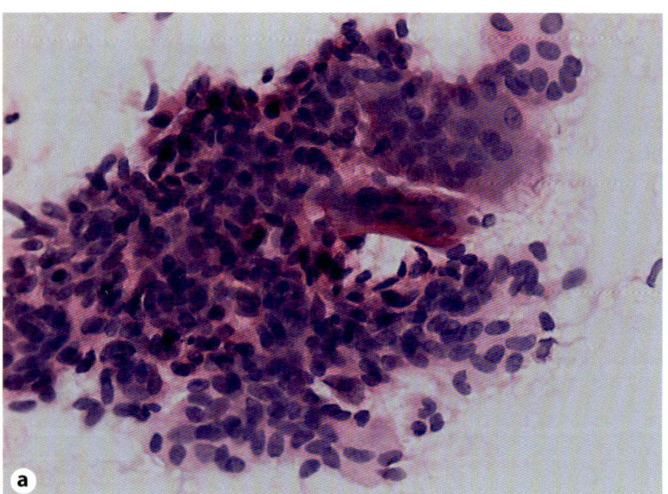

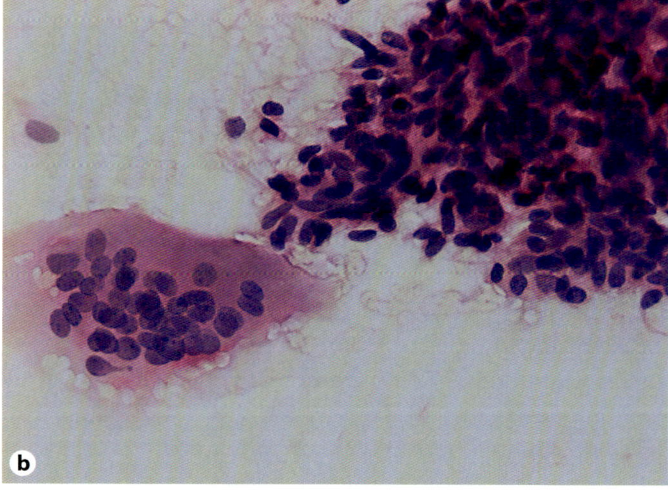

Fig. 57. As in giant cell tumours, 2 cell populations make up the smears: clustered spindly cells and multinucleated giant cells. A type-specific diagnosis depends on the radiographic features. HE, medium magnification.

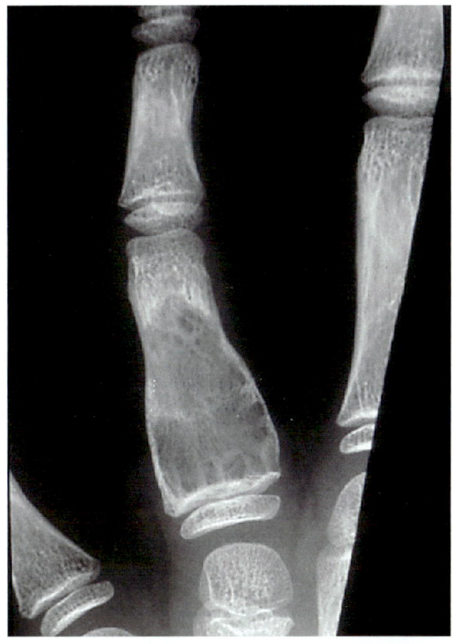

Fig. 58. Giant-cell reparative granuloma. Radiological features. PA radiograph of the forth finger. An expansile osteolytic lesion in the metaphysis and diaphysis of the proximal phalanx is seen. The cortex is thin but not destroyed. There are no calcifications within the lesion.

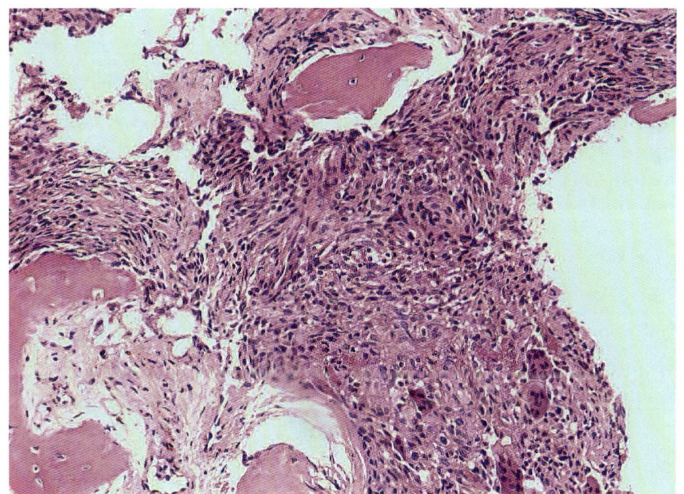

Fig. 59. Histology. This lesion is made up of fibrous tissue with clusters of spindle cells between bone trabeculae. Scattered multinucleated giant cells are present. HE, low magnification.

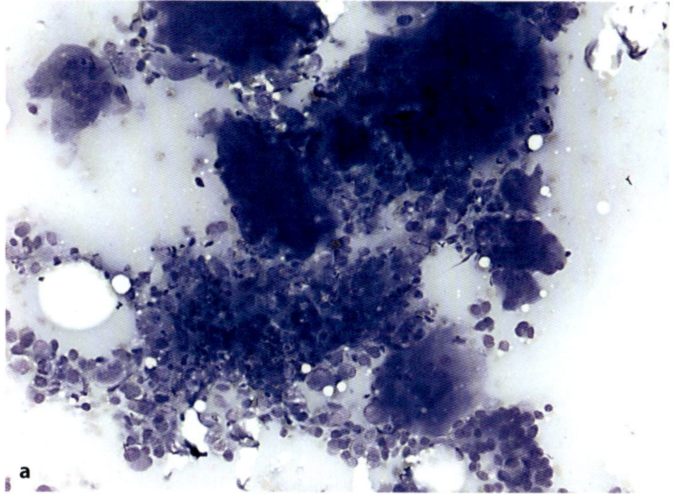

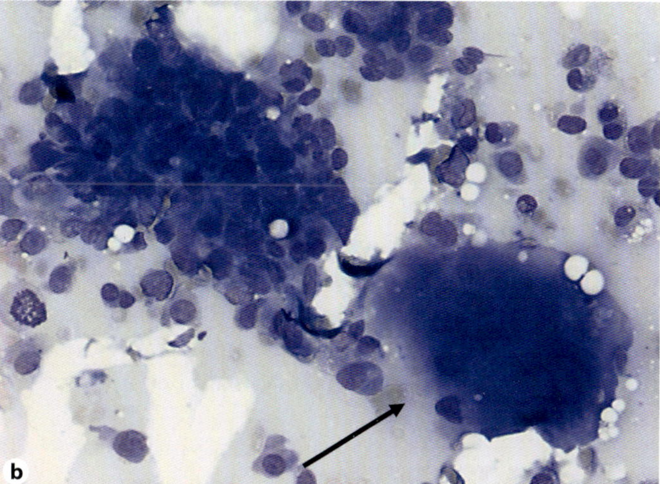

Fig. 60. a Clusters of spindly cells are mixed with multinucleated giant cells in FNA smears from the same lesion. MGG, low magnification. **b** Scattered osteoblast-like cells are seen among the spindle cells and multinucleated giant cells (arrow). MGG, high magnification.

is usually seen as reactive bone trabeculae rimmed by osteoblasts.

Cytological Features

See figure 60. There are groups or clusters of spindle cells, and multinucleated giant cells, osteoblasts and histiocytes are seen.

Differential Diagnosis

The differential diagnoses are: conventional giant-cell tumour; aneurysmal bone cyst, and brown tumour of hyperparathyroidism.

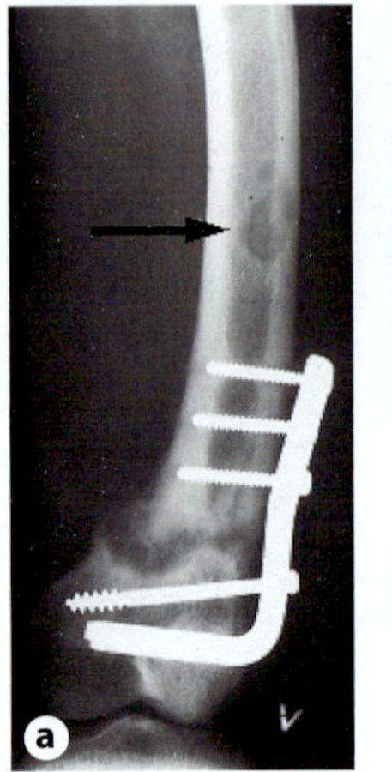

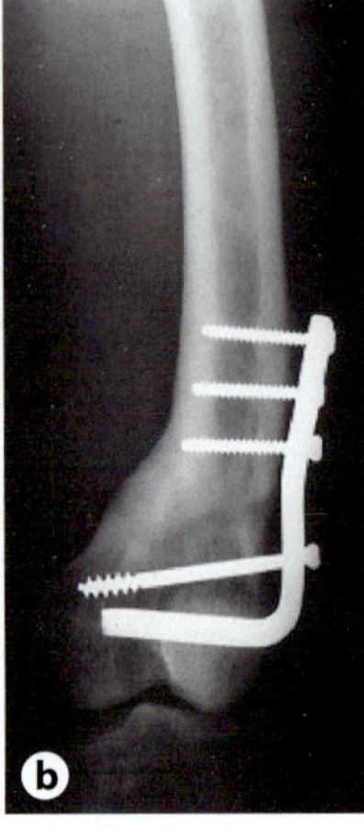

Fig. 61. Osteitis fibrosa cystica (brown tumour of hyperparathyroidism). Radiology. **a** AP radiograph of the distal femur. There is a well demarcated lytic lesion without sclerotic margins in the diaphysis (arrow). This lytic lesion represents a brown tumour secondary to parathyroid adenoma. The patient has had an osteotomy in the metaphysis fixed with a plate and screws. The osteotomy has not healed. **b** The parathyroid adenoma was resected. After 4 months, a new AP radiograph indicates that both the brown tumour and the osteotomy had healed. The bone structure is normal.

Comments
From our experience of single cases, it is difficult or impossible to cytologically distinguish reparative granuloma from giant-cell tumour and aneurysmal bone cyst in FNA smears.

Osteitis Fibrosa Cystica

One possible result of the high levels of parathyroid hormone in hyperparathyroidism is the rare tumour-like lesion osteitis fibrosa cystica, or brown tumour of hyperparathyroidism. The predilection sites for this lesion are facial and pelvic bones, ribs and femur. The site in the long bones is predominantly dia- or metaphyseal.

Radiology
See figure 61. The brown tumour is a lytic lesion, that may be well or ill defined. The lesions characteristically resolve once the cause (hyperparathyroidism) is treated.

Histopathology
Due to the increased osteoclastic bone resorption secondary to the elevated levels of parathyroid hormone, the bone trabeculae are replaced by fibrous tissue containing variable amounts of osteoclastic giant cells. More or less numerous haemosiderin-laden macrophages secondary to haemorrhage are always seen. Foci of reactive bone formation may be found.

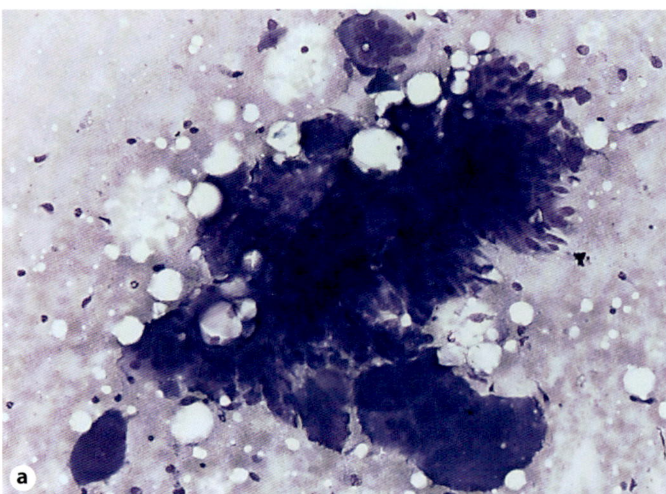

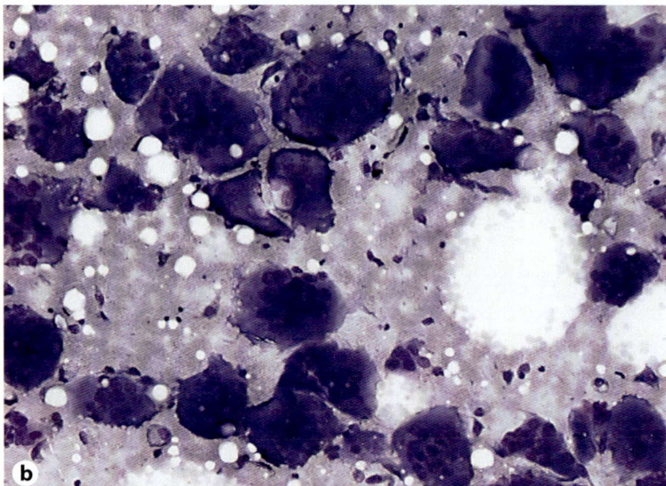

Fig. 62. b FNA smears from brown tumours are remarkably like those from giant-cell tumours: multiple multinucleated giant cells mixed with dispersed or clustered spindly cells. MGG, medium magnification.

Cytological Features
See figure 62. There are dispersed or clustered spindle cells, and variable amounts of osteoclast-like giant cells and haemosiderin-laden macrophages.

Differential Diagnosis
The differential diagnoses are: conventional giant cell tumour; aneurysmal bone cyst, and reparative giant-cell granuloma.

Comments

Brown tumours of hyperparathyroidism are infrequent and are very rarely the target for FNAC. Single case reports have been published [79, 80] and our experience is based on 1 case. In this case, the cytological findings were almost identical to those of a giant cell tumour: cohesive clusters of mononuclear spindly cells, the clusters bordered by osteoclast-like giant cells. Without knowledge of the patient's age, clinical history, site of lesion and radiographic features it may be impossible to distinguish a brown tumour of hyperparathyroidism from a giant-cell tumour in FNA smears.

Chapter 10

Rare Targets for FNAC and Diagnostic Problems with Benign Tumours/Lesions with Variable Numbers of Osteoclast-Like Giant Cells

There are several bone tumours/lesions which are only rarely targets for FNAC. In these instances, the cytological criteria used for diagnosis have been only incompletely evaluated.

Rare Targets: Metaphyseal Fibrous Defect

This metaphyseal lesion – also known as fibrous cortical defect or non-ossifying fibroma – usually occurs in the second decade and is most often an incidental finding, although a pathological fracture may be the presenting sign. The femur and the tibia are predilection sites. This lesion is virtually never seen after the age of 30.

Radiology
As a rule, a metaphyseal fibrous defect occurs on either the medial or the lateral aspect of the bone. The lesions have a characteristic appearance with a focal radiolucent area in the cortex and adjacent medullary bone. They are surrounded by a thin rim of sclerosis.

Histopathology
Metaphyseal fibrous defect is a cellular lesion composed of spindly cells with a fascicular or storiform pattern. The spindle-cell population is uniform with regular nuclei often exhibiting a prominent nucleolus. Osteoclast-like giant cells are haphazardly distributed and aggregates of siderophages and lipophages may be present. Reactive bone trabeculae with an osteoblastic rim can also be found.

Rare Targets: Fibrous Dysplasia

Fibrous dysplasia is a solitary or multifocal intramedullary lesion. The solitary (monostotic) type is most common (70–90%), 20–30% are polyostotic. Two thirds of cases are diagnosed before the age of 40 and the highest incidence is in the second decade. The most frequently affected bones are the craniofacial bones, the ribs, femur and tibia, although any bone may be involved. Common symptoms are soft tissue swelling, deformity of the affected bone and even pathological fracture. Lesions in the craniofascial bones may cause nerve damage by narrowing of the bone canals and orbit, which may cause blindness.

Radiology
In the long bones the lesions are usually expansile in the diaphysis. They are centrally or eccentrically located causing cortical thinning or local erosions. The lesions are radiolucent with a hazy appearance described as being like 'ground glass'. They are well defined, often surrounded by a rim of reactive sclerosis. Central matrix calcifications may be present, these are best seen with CT. Due to the cortical thinning, there is a risk of fracture, even after minor trauma. The lesions usually heal with age and become filled out through diffuse sclerosis.

The lesions in the craniofascial bones are radiographically radiolucent or sclerotic, or both. Sclerosis often dominates in the skull, causing expansion of the bone in an outward direction. The outer table of the vault is thus always convex.

In the spine, the radiographic characteristics are the same as in other locations. In the spine the polyostotic type of involvement is more common than the monostotic. As in other sites the cortex is thinned and the vertebral body may collapse after minor trauma.

Histopathology
Fibrous dysplasia is a fibro-osseous lesion made up of a more or less cellular fibrous stroma containing a variable amount of irregularly arranged bony trabeculae, usually without an osteoblastic rim. The bony trabeculae are often described as being similar to Chinese characters. Osteoclast-like giant cells are commonly present.

Comments
These 2 lesions are very seldom the targets for FNAC as their radiographic findings are rather distinctive, and their cytological features almost unknown. Clusters of spindle cells together with osteoclast-like giant cells and the presence of foamy macrophages were described in 1 reported case of metaphyseal fibrous defect [81]. The cytological findings in 1 case of fibrous dysplasia have also been recorded. The smears contained blood, osteoclast-like giant cells and tissue fragments, probably representing woven bone [82]. Presumably, the only indication for FNAC is when the presenting symptom is a pathological fracture.

Rare Targets: Adamantinoma

Adamantinoma is an extremely rare tumour, mainly seen in the tibia and occasionally in the fibula. According to Czerniak et al. [83], there are 2 subtypes of adamantinoma, classical and differentiated. Classic adamantinoma is a tumour of adults, while differentiated adamantinoma occurs in the first 2 decades. The classic type may show cortical destruction and involve soft tissue while differentiated adamantinoma is an intracortical tumour.

Radiology
The adamantinoma is most often located eccentrically in the anterior aspect of the cortex and medulla. It is expansile, often well defined with reactive bone sclerosis and small radiolucent foci.

Histopathology
In classic adamantinoma, epithelial-like cells predominate, with tubular, basaloid, spindly and squamoid patterns being described [84]. The epithelial formations are embedded in a various amount of fibrous stroma. The differentiated type, on the other hand, is similar to osteo-fibrous dysplasia, containing small rests of epithelial formations.

Cytological Features of Classic Adamantinoma
There is a predominant population of bland spindle-shaped cells. Cohesive clusters or groups of rounded epithelial cells with bland chromatin and small nucleoli are also seen.

Comments
Adamantimona is an extremely rare primary bone tumour and only single case reports of FNAC of adamantinoma have been published [85, 86]. The clue to a cytological diagnosis is the double cell population of spindle-shaped mesenchymal and epithelial cells. A FNAC diagnosis of adamantinoma must be based on the combined evaluation of clinical and radiographic data and cytomorphology.

Benign Bone Tumours/Lesions: Diagnostic Problems with Variable Numbers of Osteoclast-Like Giant Cells

It is obvious from previous chapters that the many benign tumours and lesions featuring more or less numerous osteoclast-like multinucleated giant cells in the fine needle aspirate smears constitute a diagnostic challenge for the cytopathologist.

The cytological features of many of those entities are very similar, precluding a type-specific diagnosis based only on the cytological findings. In most cases, however, it is possible to define the lesion as a benign tumour/lesion with numerous giant cells. A type-specific diagnosis is only possible when knowledge of clinical and radiographic findings are combined with the cytological features.

Table 8. Benign bone tumours/lesions exhibiting osteoclast-like giant cells in aspirate smears

Osteoblastoma
Chondroblastoma
Chondromyxoid fibroma
Giant-cell tumour
Aneurysmal bone cyst
Giant-cell reparative granuloma
Osteitis fibrosa cystica (brown tumour of hyperparathyroidism)
Fibrous dysplasia
Fibrous metaphyseal defect (non-ossifying fibroma)

Table 9. Summary of main diagnostic criteria in benign tumours/lesions exhibiting osteoclast-like giant cells

Tumour/lesion	Age, years	Predilection sites	Radiology	Cytology
Osteoblastoma	10–30	spine, sacrum, proximal and distal femur	well circumscribed, thinning of cortex, calcifications	osteoblasts, osteoclasts, groups of spindle cells
Chondroblastoma	20–30	epiphysis of long tubular bones	osteolytic, sharply demarcated, thin sclerotic rim (calcifications)	chondroid matrix fragments with chondroblasts, often indented nuclei ('coffee-bean' nuclei)
Chondromyxoid fibroma	10–30	femur, tibia metaphysis	osteolytic, elongated, eccentric lesion	myxoid matrix, cartilaginous fragments, spindly cells, spindly and chondroid cells often pleomorphic
Giant cell tumour	20–40	epiphyses of long tubular bones	blown-up lytic lesion	clustered mononuclear cells, numerous giant cells
Aneurysmal bone cyst	10–25	metaphyses in long tubular bones		haemorrhagic smears, spindle cells, giant cells, histiocytes
Giant-cell reparative granuloma	10–30	craniofascial bones, small bones of hands and feet	lytic lesion	clusters of mononuclear spindle cells, giant cells, histiocytes (osteoblasts)
Osteitis fibrosa cystica/ brown tumour of hyperparathyroidism	40–70	fascial and pelvic bones, femur, ribs, dia- and metaphyseal lesions		clusters of mononuclear cells, numerous giant cells
Fibrous metaphyseal defect/ non-ossifying fibroma	10–20	femur, tibia	eccentric lytic lesion	spindle cells, giant cells[1]
Fibrous dysplasia	10–20	craniofascial bones, ribs, femur, tibia	central lytic defect	giant cells, bone fragments[1]

[1] Cytology has not been sufficiently evaluated at present.

The various benign entities featuring multinucleated giant cells are presented in table 8, and a summary of pertinent diagnostic data are in table 9.

Clinically, the most important diagnostic pitfalls are to misdiagnose an osteoclast-rich osteosarcoma as a conventional giant-cell tumour, and to diagnose a chondromyxoid fibroma as a chondrosarcoma.

Chapter 11

Lymphohaematopoetic and Histiocytic Tumours

Solitary Plasmacytoma of Bone

Solitary plasmacytoma of bone is a bone lesion composed of neoplastic plasma cells identical to plasma cells in myeloma. Solitary plasmacytoma of bone occurs predominantly in elderly patients (60–70 years of age) and is rare before the age of 40. The lesion is most common in bones with active haematopoesis, such as vertebrae, ribs, the pelvic bones, skull and femur. Importantly, light chain restriction is not always found and patients with solitary plasmacytoma do not always have M protein in the blood or urine.

Radiology
See figure 63. Solitary plasmacytoma of bone is often a well circumscribed, expansile lytic lesion within the bone marrow and with a geographic pattern. The overlying cortical bone is often thin and a cortical perforation may be seen on CT or MRI. The tumour often looks benign on plain radiography.

Histopathology
As in myeloma, the neoplastic plasma cells show variable features, which range from those indistinguishable from normal plasma cells to pleomorphic or anaplastic forms. Bi-nucleated and multinucleated plasma cells are also part of the morphological spectrum.

Cytological Features
See figure 64. The smears are often haemorrhagic with abundant plasma cells. Cells are predominantly dispersed but small clusters of loosely cohesive cells may be seen. There is variable cell differentiation from normal-looking plasma cells to highly pleomorphic (bi- or multinucleated) cells. Cells with plasmablastic morphology (immunoblast-like cells with prominent central nucleoli) occasionaly predominate.

Differential Diagnosis
The differential diagnoses are: large B-cell lymphoma of immunoblastic type; reactive benign plasmacytosis. and metastasis of anaplastic carcinoma.

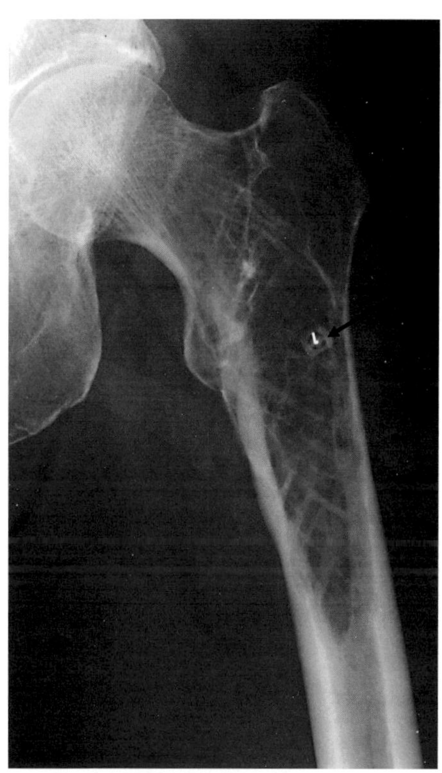

Fig. 63. Solitary plasmacytoma. Radiological features. PA radiograph of the left femur. An extensive osteolytic destruction from the lateral aspect of the femoral neck to several cm below the lesser trochanter is present. There is no cortical destruction. Arrow indicates needle track.

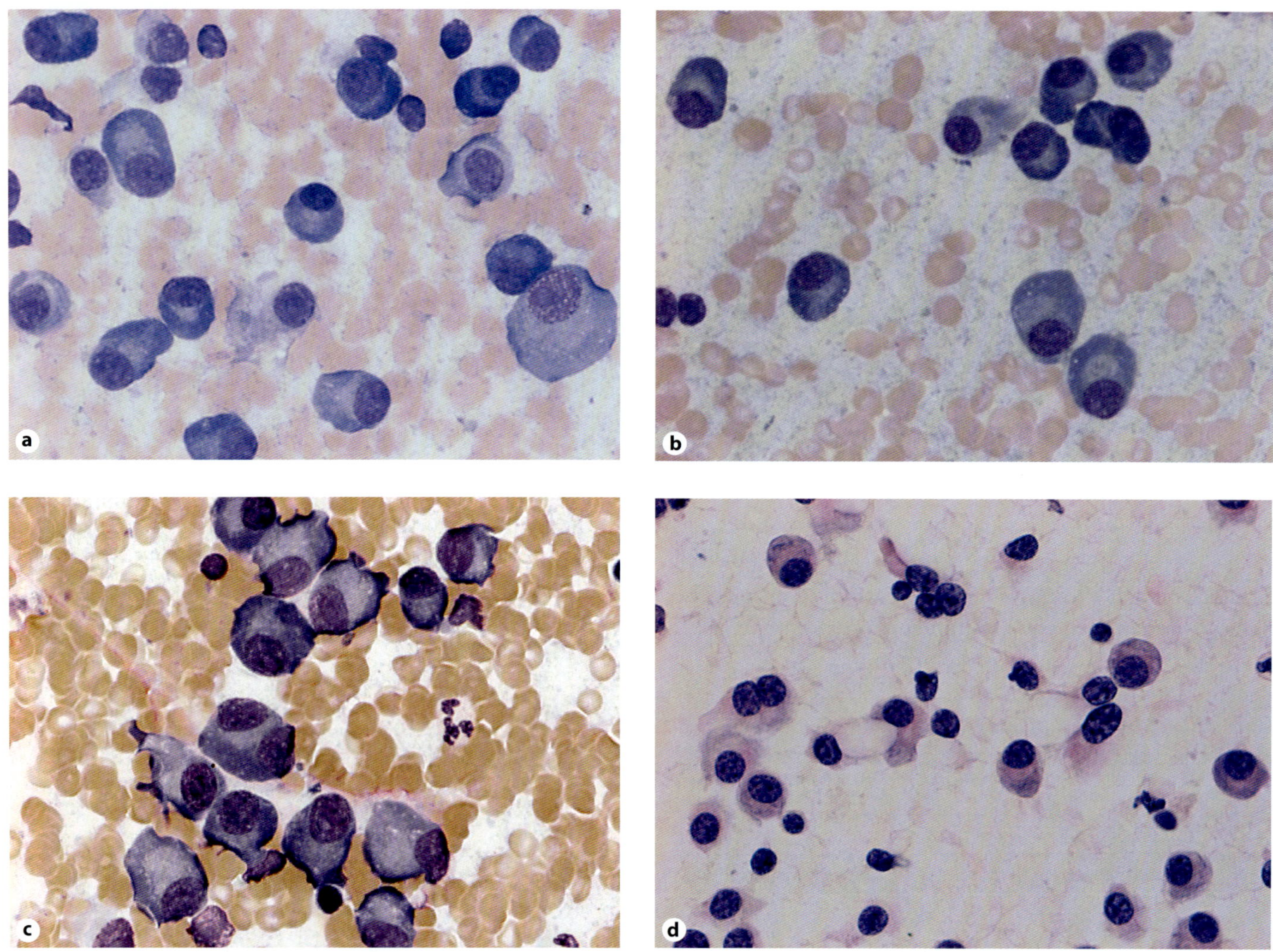

Fig. 64. Smears from solitary plasmacytomas often show similar features. Smears from 4 different cases are shown. Moderately atypical plasma cells are present in a more or less haemorrhagic background. **a–c** MGG, medium magnification. **d** HE, medium magnification.

Comments

Due to the thin, at times perforated cortical bone, plasmacytomas are most often easy to needle and the yield is rich. The diagnostic criteria are a solitary bone lesion and no evidence of plasmacytosis in the bone marrow. Complete radiographic investigation of the skeleton is thus necessary. It is not possible to distinguish a reactive plasmacytosis from plasmacytoma in haemorrhagic aspirates featuring a low number of normal-looking plasma cells. Likewise, the diagnosis is difficult when the sample contains a prominent admixture of normal bone marrow cells.

Osteoblasts resemble plasma cells, while reactive osteoblasts may be mistaken for atypical plasma cells. However, the cytoplasmic 'Hof' is paranuclear in plasma cells.

Poorly differentiated (anaplastic) plasmacytoma features highly atypical tumour cells with variable amounts of cytoplasm and often nucleolated nuclei. Often there are no signs of a cytoplasmic Hof (fig. 65).

The neoplastic plasma cells express monotypic immunoglobulin, and in most cases it is possible to diagnose a light chain restriction in cell block or cytospin preparations (fig. 66). The neoplastic plasma cells, including the pleomorphic and atypical forms, express CD138 and CD79A but not CD20.

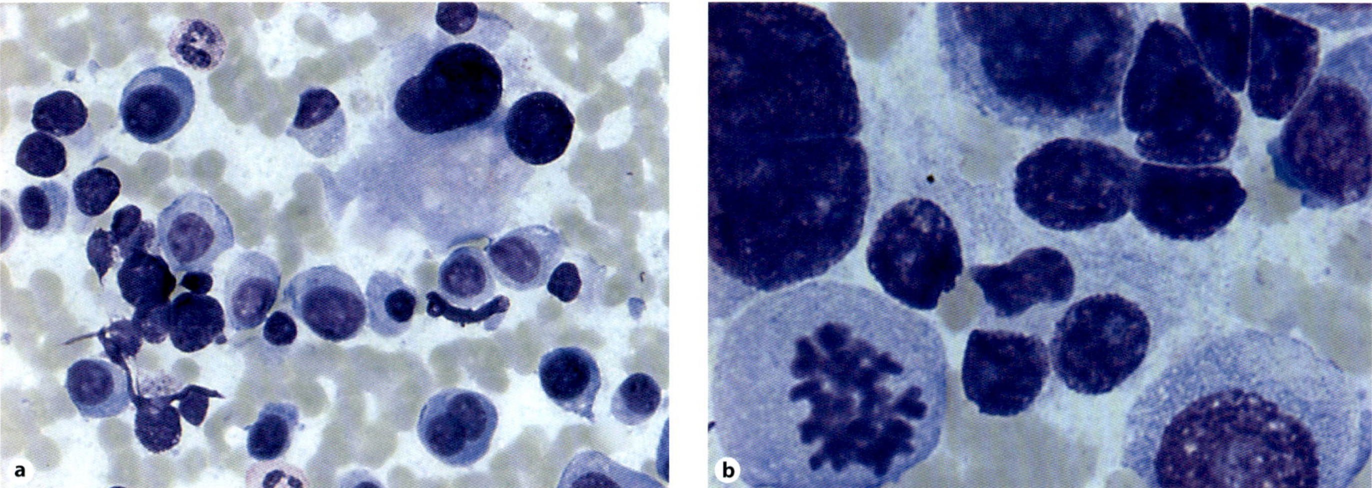

Fig. 65. In poorly differentiated, anaplastic plasmacytoma the cellular and nuclear atypia is marked and the pleomorphic plasma cells are difficult to diagnose as such. **a** MGG, medium magnification. **b** MGG, high magnification.

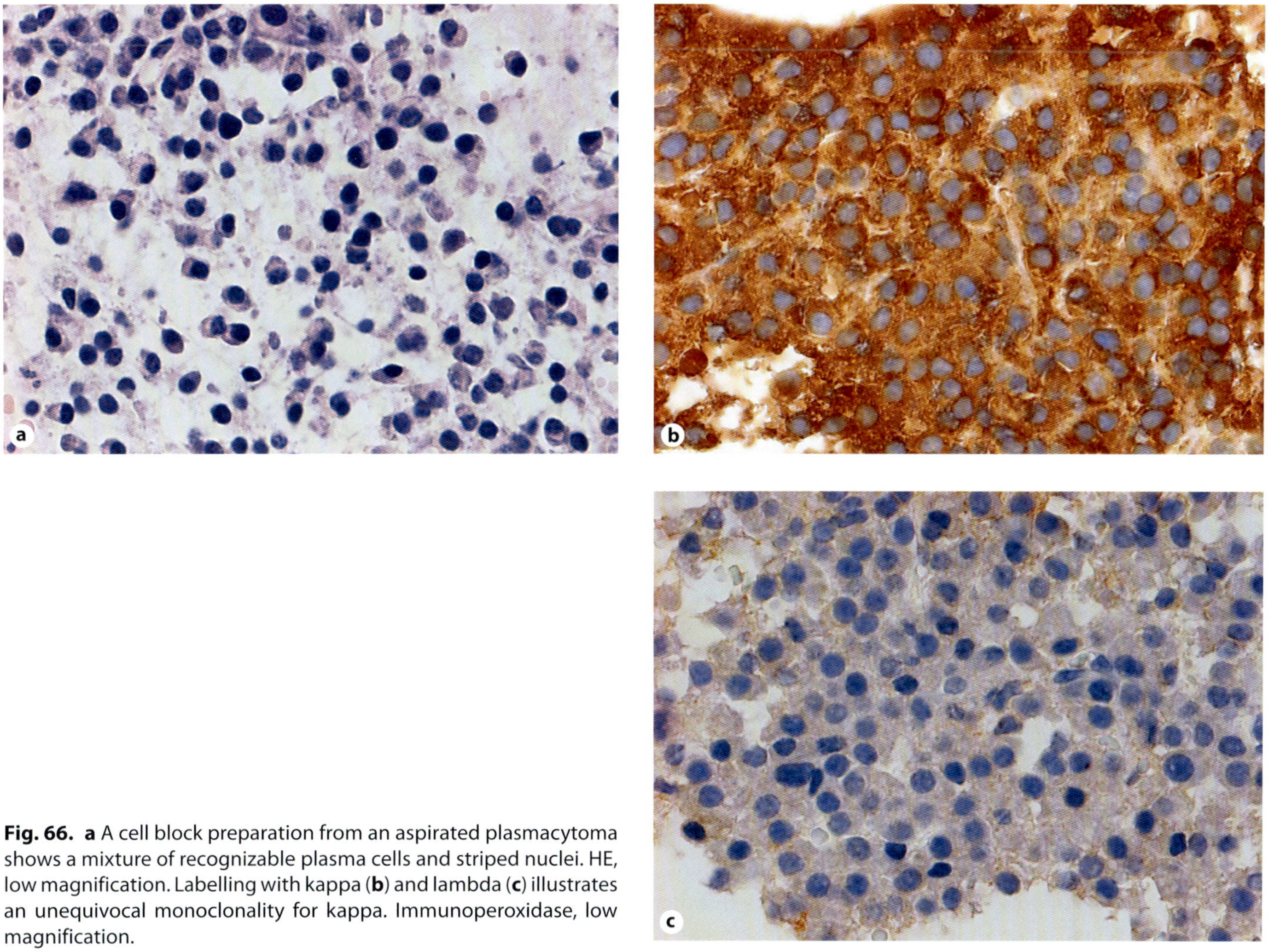

Fig. 66. a A cell block preparation from an aspirated plasmacytoma shows a mixture of recognizable plasma cells and striped nuclei. HE, low magnification. Labelling with kappa (**b**) and lambda (**c**) illustrates an unequivocal monoclonality for kappa. Immunoperoxidase, low magnification.

Primary Lymphoma of Bone

Primary lymphoma of bone is a very rare lesion which is defined as a lymphoma in a solitary bone with no signs of other skeletal or non-skeletal sites within 6 months after onset of symptoms. Primary lymphoma of bone comprise approximately 3–7% of all malignant bone tumours. A primary bone lymphoma can appear at any age but most patients are over 45 years of age. Certain subtypes, such as precursor (lymphoblastic) lymphoma and anaplastic large-cell lymphoma, may arise in children and young adults. The majority of lymphomas occur in the long bones, followed by the pelvic bones and the vertebral column.

Radiology
The radiological findings are non-characteristic. There are often osteolytic lesions with moth-eaten or permeative bone destruction. Cortical destruction indicates a soft tissue component. Periosteitis may also occur.

Histopathology
The vast majority of lymphomas are aggressive B-cell lymphomas (diffuse large B-cell lymphoma). Lymphoplasmacytic lymphoma, precursor lymphoma and anaplastic large-cell lymphoma have also been reported [87–89]. Primary Hodgkin lymphoma in bone is extremely rare. At the Mayo Clinic only 5 patients with primary Hodgkin lymphoma were identified during the years 1927–1996 [90]. Both histopathological and cytological criteria for diagnosis are the same as for non-osseous lymphoma. The cytodiagnosis of primary bone lymphoma has been reported [91–93].

Differential Diagnosis
The differential diagnoses are: classical Ewing's sarcoma; immunoblastic or plasmablastic variants of plasmocytoma; granulocytic sarcoma; metastatic small-cell undifferentiated carcinoma, and osteosarcoma (anaplastic large-cell lymphoma).

Comments
In addition to a few cases of diffuse large B-cell lymphoma, single cases of precursor lymphoma and anaplastic large cell lymphoma are recorded in our files (fig. 67–69). When a non-Hodgkin lymphoma is a diagnostic alternative, ancillary techniques are indispensable to reach a correct diagnosis.

The same methods are used as in cases of non-osseous lymphoma. Our experience with flow cytometric immunophenotyping is favourable. Lin et al. [91] and Söderlund et al. [92] have relied successfully on immunocytochemistry.

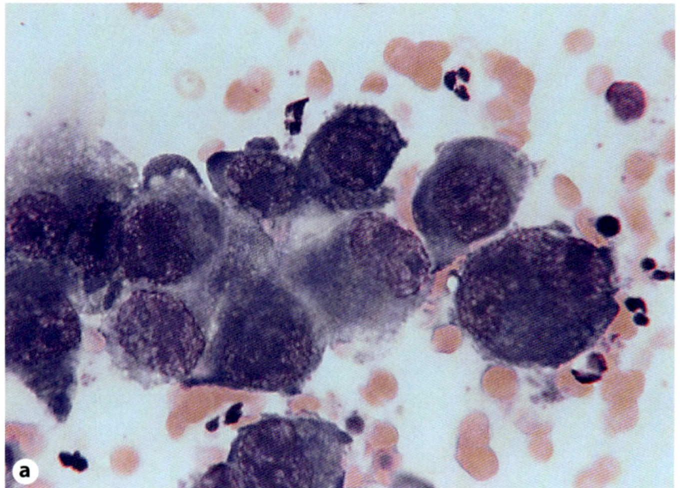

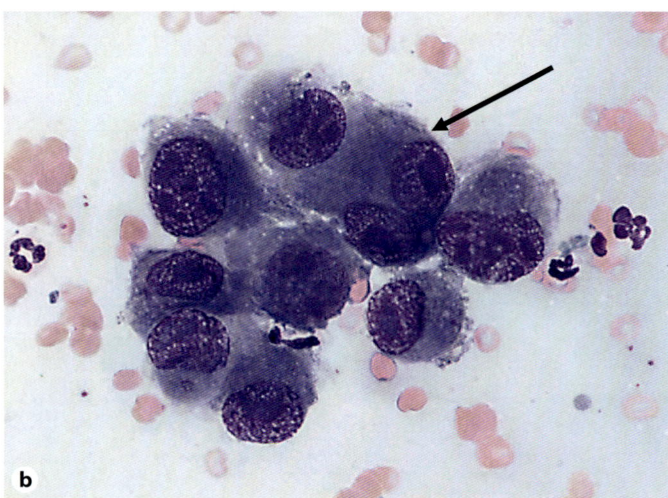

Fig. 67. a, b Primary anaplastic large cell lymphoma of the femur. Clusters of large cytoplasm-rich cells with rounded nuclei exhibiting prominent nucleoli. Note the Reed-Sternberg-like binucleated cell in **b** (arrow). MGG, high magnification.

It is recommended not to forget to include terminal deoxynucleotidyl transferase in the antibody panel when a precursor lymphoma is suspected, and to include CD30, EMA and Alk-1 to reliably diagnose anaplastic large-cell lymphoma.

Langerhans Cell Histiocytosis

Langerhans cell histiocytosis – also known as eosinophilic granuloma or histiocytosis X – is a localized or systemic proliferation of Langerhans cells.

Most frequent sites are bones and skin. Langerhans cell histiocytosis may appear at any age but the majority of

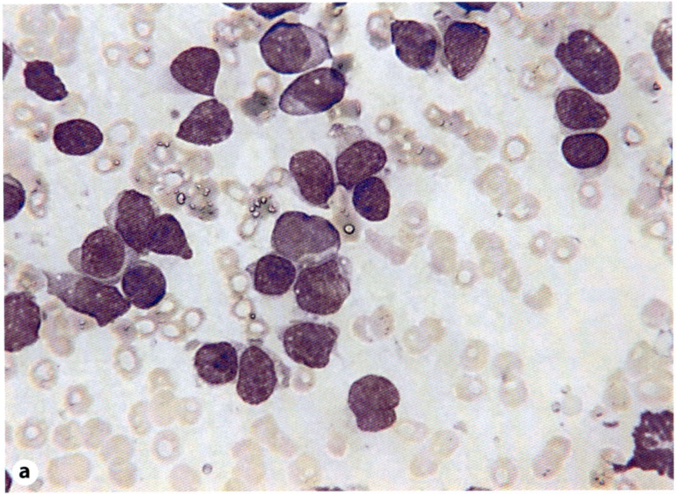

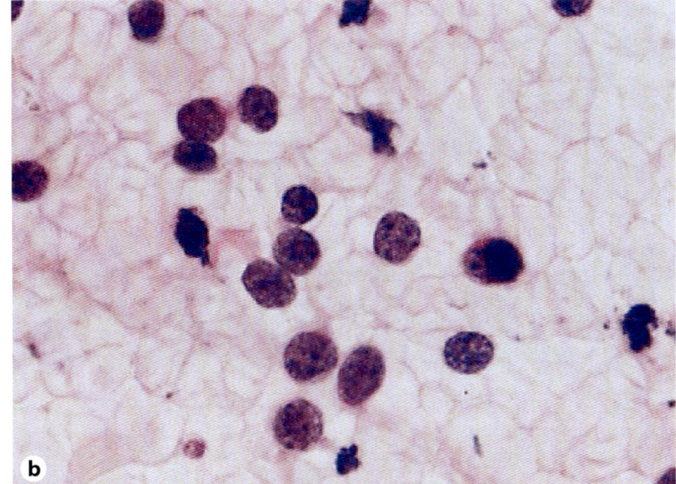

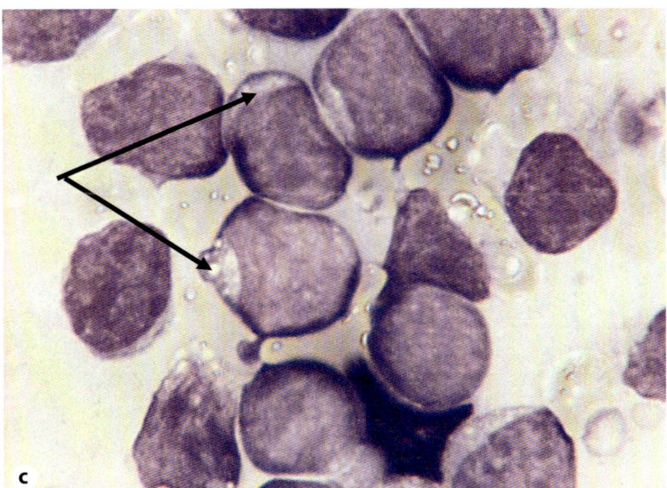

Fig. 68. Primary precursor B-cell lymphoma of the sacrum. **a**, **b** Medium-sized lymphoid cells with irregular nuclei and scanty cytoplasm. The chromatin texture is finely granular and nucleoli insignificant or lacking. MGG, medium magnification (a). HE, medium magnification (**b**). **c** A typical feature in many precursor lymphoma cells in FNA smears is the presence of a pale paranuclear area in the cytoplasm (arrow). MGG, high magnification.

cases occur in children between 5 and 10 years of age. The bone lesions might be solitary (most common) or multiple. Langerhans cell histiocytosis may arise in any bone.

The skull, femur and humerus are the commonest sites in children, and the skull, pelvic bones and ribs in adults.

Radiology
See figure 70. The lesions are often well defined and lytic, as exemplified in the skull and pelvic bones. Sometimes a central radiodense focus is present within the skull lesions, called 'button' sequestrum. In the spine the destruction often leads to a flattened vertebral body, a 'vertebra plana'.

Lesions in the long bones are initially well defined and radiolucent, but with further growth they encroach on the cortical bone which may lead to periosteal new bone formation. Lesions in the ribs may cause a pathological fracture.

Histopathology
Langerhans cells are arranged in non-cohesive clusters or sheets or appear as single cells. They have an abundant faintly eosinophilic cytoplasm. The nuclei are ovoid or characteristically grooved, polylobated or indented. So called 'coffee-bean' nuclei are not uncommon. The chromatin texture is bland and the nucleoli inconspicuous. Binucleated and multinucleated cells are commonly observed. The mitotic rate is generally low. In addition to the Langerhans cells, inflammatory cells are part of the lesion. Variable numbers of eosinophilic leucocytes, lymphocytes, histiocytes and osteoclast-like giant cells are present and eventually plasma cells. The Langerhans cells stain for S-100 protein and CD1A and feature so-called Birbeck's granulae at electron microscopic examination.

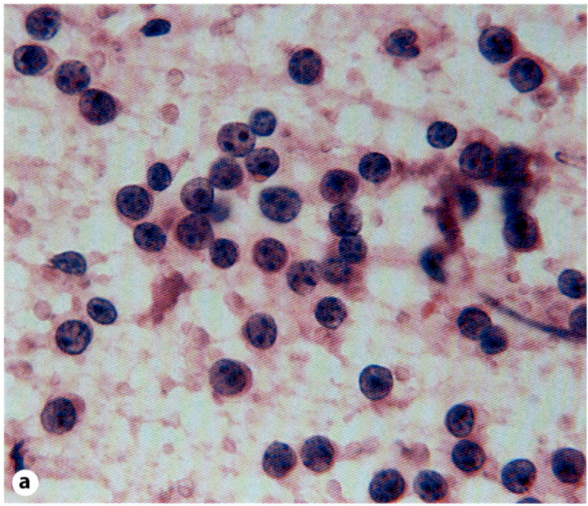

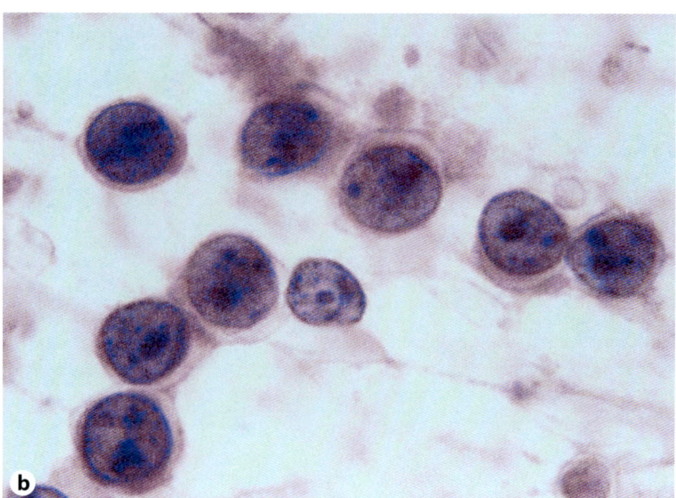

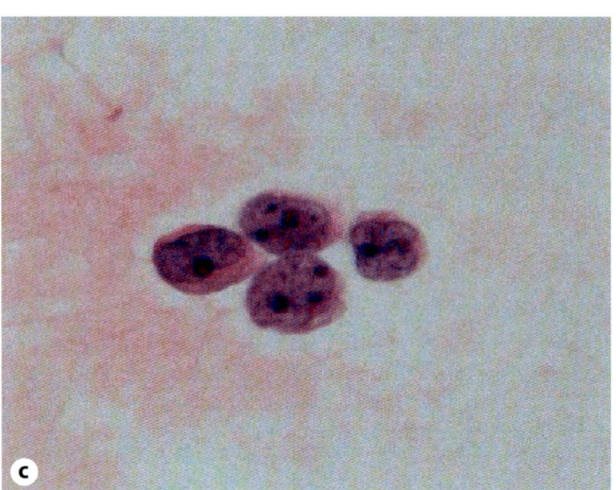

Fig. 69. Primary large B-cell lymphoma of the femur. **a** Dispersed rather uniform rounded tumour cells with scanty cytoplasm on a haemorraghic background. HE, low magnification. **b** The cells have rounded nuclei with prominent nucleoli often near the nuclear membrane. HE, high magnification. **c** The typical features of centroblasts (membrane-near nucleoli) are even more evident in a cytospin preparation from the aspirate to be used for immunocytochemistry. HE, high magnification.

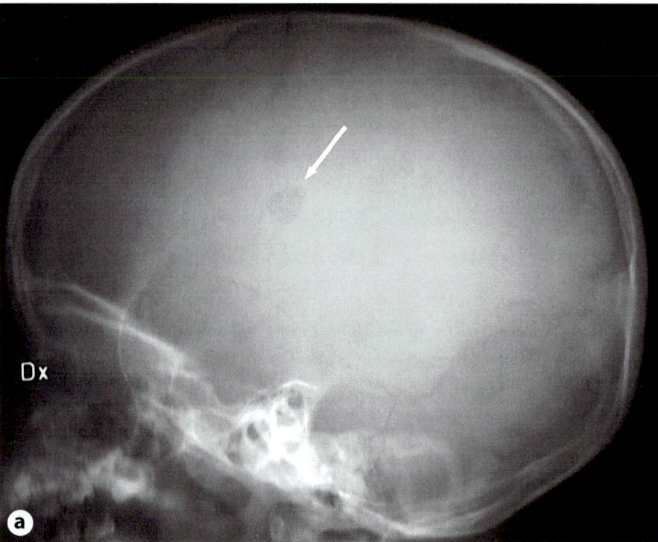

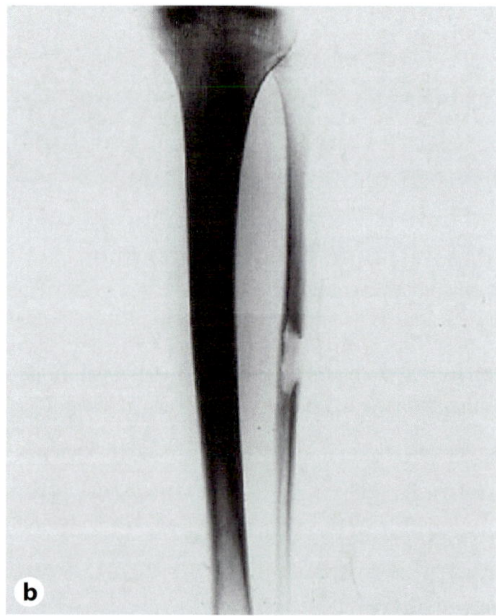

Fig. 70. Langerhans-cell histiocytosis. Radiology. **a** Lateral radiograph of the skull. Small lytic lesion in the parietal bone (arrow). **b** AP radiograph of the lower leg. A well defined lytic lesion in the diaphysis of the fibula.

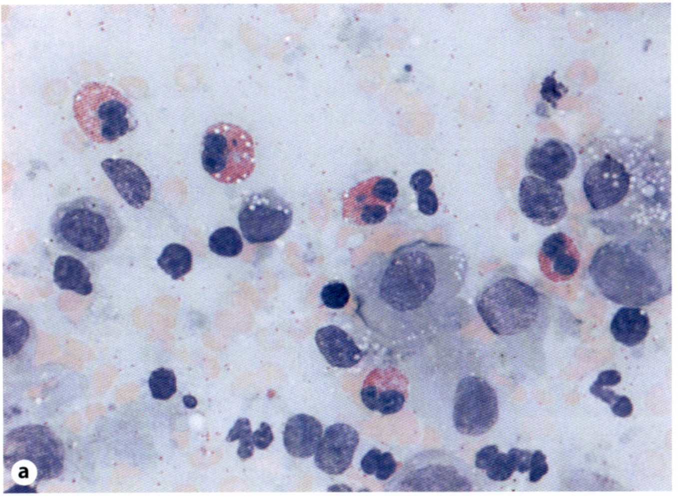

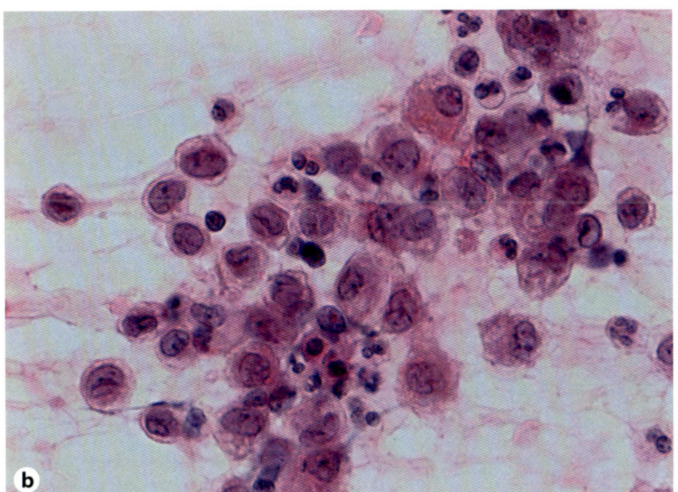

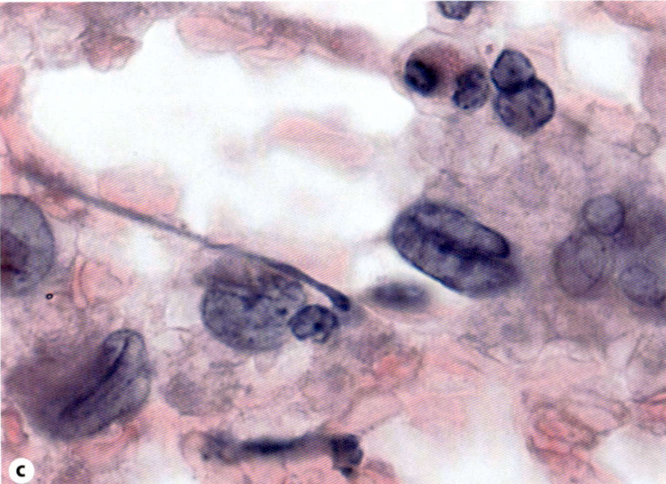

Fig. 71. **a** Histiocytes with abundant cytoplasm and rounded or ovoid nuclei mixed with neutrophilic and eosinophilic leucocytes. MGG, medium magnification. **b, c** Lobulated or 'coffee-bean' nuclei are typical features of the histiocytes in Langerhans-cell histiocytosis. **b** HE, medium magnification. **c** HE, high magnification.

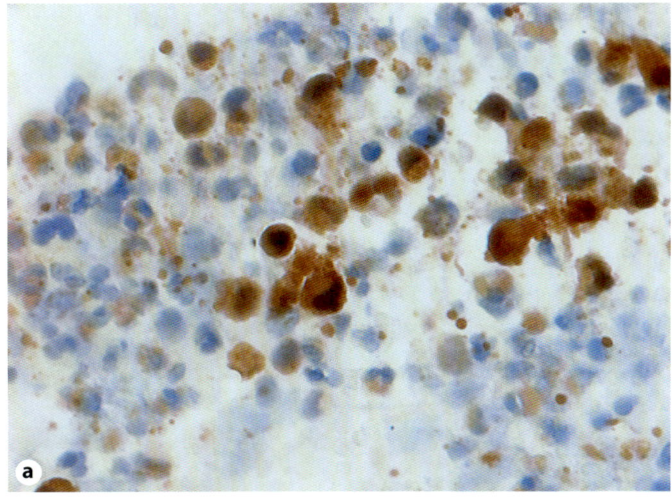

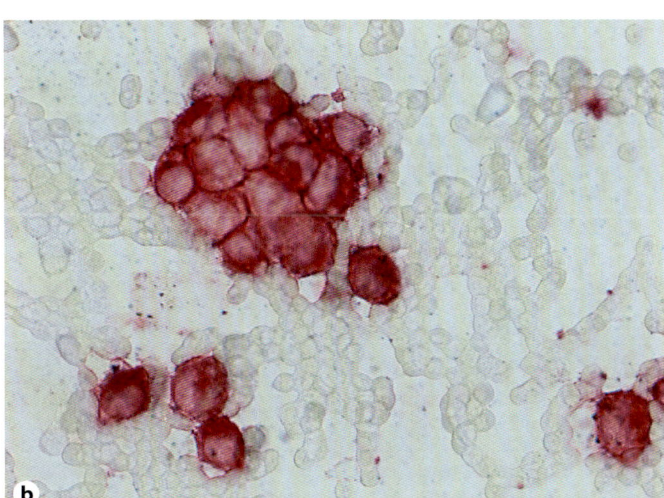

Fig. 72. S-100 protein and CD1a are markers for Langerhans cells. **a** Cell block preparation, S-100 protein, immunoperoxidase, medium magnification. **b** Cytospin preparation, CD1a, medium magnification.

Cytological Features
See figure 71. Histiocytes (Langerhans cells) appear with ovoid, reniform or lobulated nuclei. Longitudinal grooves ('coffee-bean' nuclei), bland chromatin and small nucleoli are typical nuclear features and cytoplasm is abundant. Numbers of eosinophils, neutrophils and lymphocytes vary. Binucleated and multinucleated histiocytes are most often present.

Differential Diagnosis
The differential diagnosis is non-specific osteomyelitis.

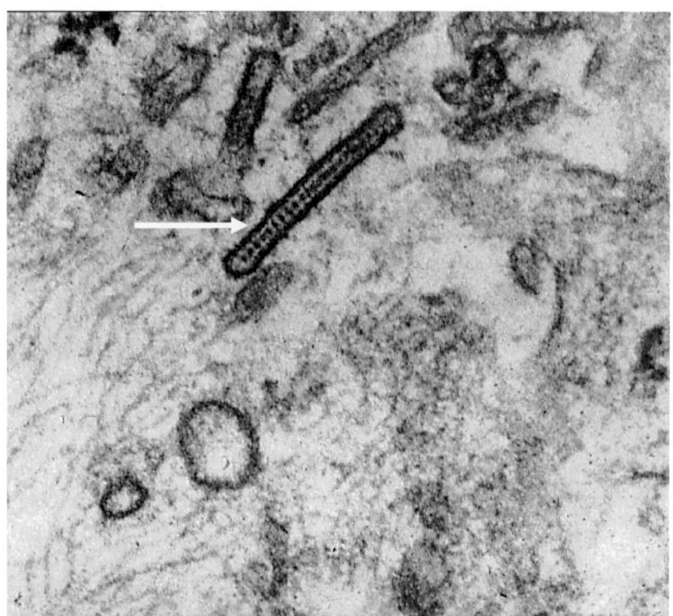

Fig. 73. Part of an aspirate prepared for electron microscopic examination. Typical Birbeck's granulae (arrow).

Comments

The cytological features of Langerhans cell histiocytosis have been described in several publications [94–97]. It has been proposed that the a correct diagnosis can be established on routinely stained smears correlated with clinical and radiographic data in a majority of cases [95]. S-100 protein as well as CD1A are markers for Langerhans cells (fig. 72). However, according to the Histiocyte Society, a definitive diagnosis should be based on morphology and histochemical expression of CD1A or the presence of Birbeck's granulae on electron microscopic examination (fig. 73).

Chapter 12

Inflammatory Lesions

Non-Specific Osteomyelitis

Most cases of osteomyelitis are of bacterial origin and staphylococci are the most common agent. Anaerobic osteomyelitis is much less common. In most cases, infection originates in another site and spreads directly from post-traumatic or operative infections. A proportion of osteomyelitis patients suffer from peripheral vascular disease, especially diabetes. Approximately 20% of cases are haematogenous, with skin, urinary and respiratory infections thought to predispose to osteomyelitis. Although acute haematogenous osteomyelitis may occur at any age, patients are usually under 15 years old. The long bones are those most commonly affected.

Radiology
See figure 74. Acute osteomyelitis is not a radiological diagnosis in the first stage. Initially the inflammatory reaction is best seen with MRI as bone marrow oedema. Bone scintigraphy has a 2-stage reaction pattern. During the first 1 or 2 days there is a 'cold spot' due to suppression of the normal osteoblastic activity caused by the oedema, later there is an increased osteoblastic activity with increased uptake within the osteomyelitic area. After 3–7 days, bone destruction may be seen on plain radiography. The destruction is most often lytic and of permeative type, and as a rule is accompanied by a periosteal reaction. Radiologically, it cannot be differentiated from a malignant bone tumour. An abscess (Brodie's abscess) appears in the subacute stage, surrounded with sclerosis of variable degree. The Brodie's abscess is well demarcated and is of geographic appearance. However, extensions from the abscess towards the cortical surface or an adjacent growth plate are seen on CT. In the chronic stage, the bone is often sclerotic, although a lytic pattern may be seen with 1 or several sclerotic sequestra (islands of dead bone) within the lesion.

Histopathology
Bone destruction in the form of bone resorption and bone necrosis and an inflammatory infiltrate are the typical features. In acute osteomyelitis the bone marrow is replaced by neutrophils, in the subacute stage there is an admixture of plasma cells and lymphocytes besides the neutrophils.

Cytological Features of Acute Osteomyelitis
See figure 75. There is often abundant material predominantly composed of neutrophils, with histiocytes and necrotic debris also seen.

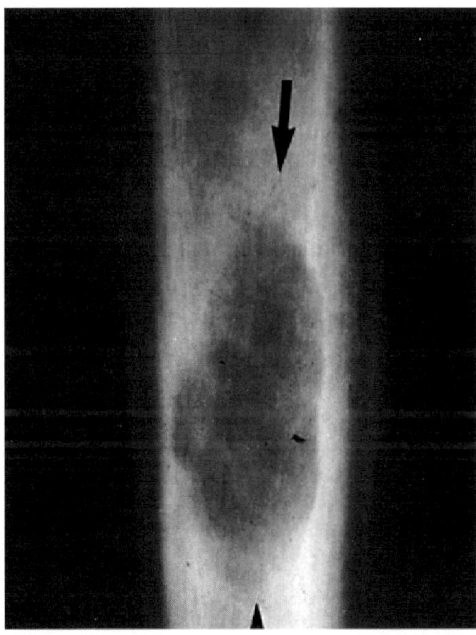

Fig. 74. Acute osteomyelitis. Radiology. Magnified detail of a plain lateral radiograph of the tibia. There is a relatively well demarcated lytic lesion centrally in the bone marrow (arrows). Dorsally there is minor cortical erosion. The lesion has a non-characteristic appearance and might represent either a benign lesion, such as osteomyelitis, or a malignant tumour.

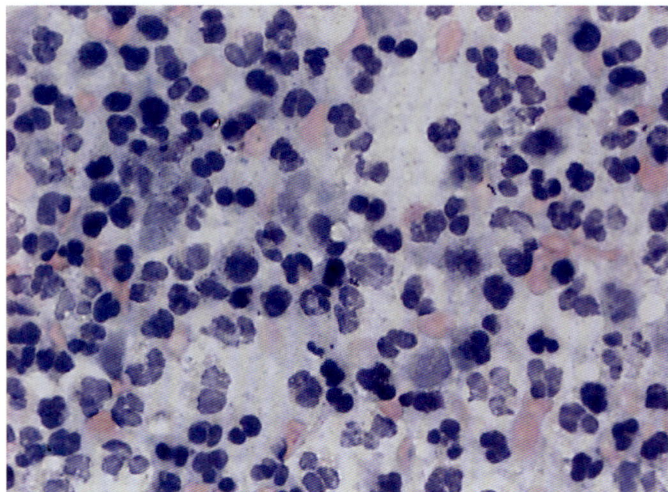

Fig. 75. Smears from non-specific acute osteomyelitis most often look like pus, with an abundance of neutrophils and necrotic debris. MGG, high magnification.

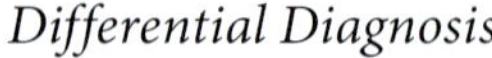

Differential Diagnosis
The differential diagnosis is: Langerhans cell histiocytosis.

Comments
As described above, the bone destruction in acute osteomyelitis is radiologically not possible to differentiate from a malignant bone tumour, in particular Ewing´s sarcoma in teenagers. In these cases FNAC is an important diagnostic tool as the abundant aspirate from an acute osteomyelitis looks like pus from any other site and is cytologically easy to distinguish from malignancy. Perhaps the most important part of the FNA is to save some of the aspirate material for culture (aerobic and anaerobic). When the inflammatory infiltrate is mixed and includes histiocytes, plasma cells and lymphocytes, Langerhans cell histiocytosis is a diagnostic pitfall as the presence of eosinophils is variable in Langerhans cell histiocytosis.

Tuberculous Osteomyelitis

Tuberculous osteomyelitis is caused by haematogenous spread from the lungs. Although it may occur in any bone, the vertebrae are the most common sites, followed by the pelvic bones and the knee.

Radiology
The initial radiographic pattern of tuberculous osteomyelitis is similar to pyogenic infections described above. Later, tuberculous granulomatous tissue and caseous necrosis may cause cyst-like, circumscribed lesions surrounded by sclerotic bone. Sequestra are uncommon.

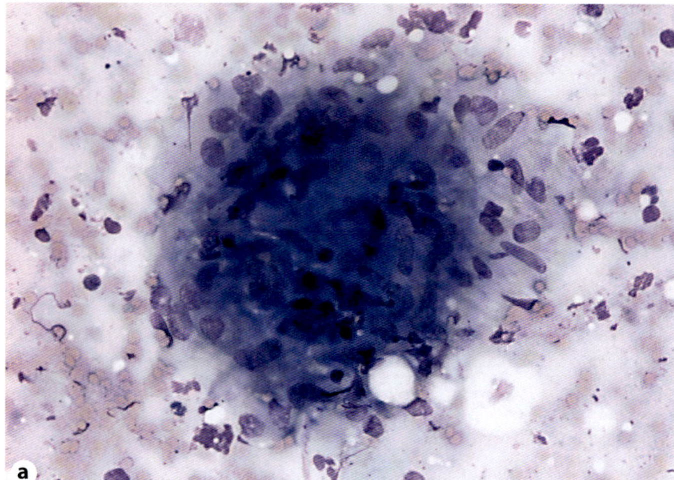

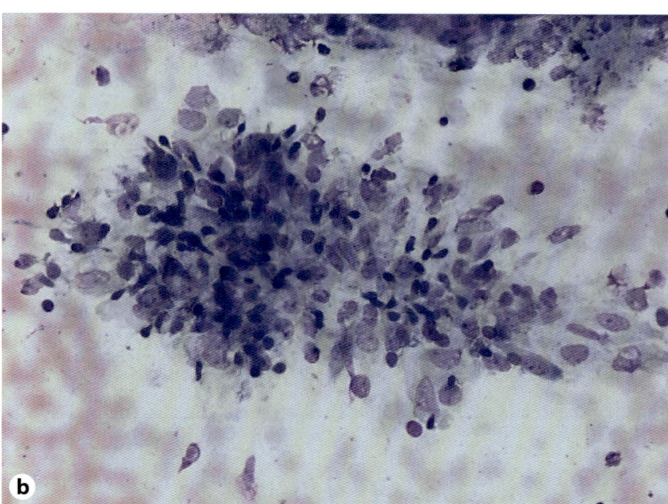

Fig. 76. Tuberculous osteomyelitis. Epithelioid cell granulomas. Clusters of moderately cohesive cells with pale reniform nuclei and poorly demarcated cytoplasm. MGG, medium magnification.

Histopathology
Characteristic findings are destruction of the vertebrae with typical necrotizing epithelioid cell granuloma.

Cytologically, the granulomas have the same appearance as epithelioid cell granulomas in lymphnodes or in other sites (fig. 76). In our experience of single cases of vertebral tuberculous osteomyelitis, the granulomas were rather easy to diagnose. They were more or less cohesive clusters of epithelioid-like cells with pale, reniform or boomerang-like nuclei and abundant poorly demarcated cytoplasm. Giant cells of Langerhans type were difficult find in our cases.

Chapter 13

Bone Metastases

Metastatic Cancer

This is the commonest malignant bone tumour. The true incidence of malignant tumours metastatizing to bone is not known. Approximately 50% of patients with malignant tumours develop metastases and half of them occur in the skeleton. In Sweden, there are roughly 40,000 new cases of malignant tumours each year and about 10,000 of these patients are thought to develop skeletal metastases. Although any bone can be affected, metastatic bone disease is mainly found in bones with active bone marrow, such as the vertebrae, pelvic bones, sternum, ribs and proximal femur. Any malignant tumours can metastatize to the skeleton but approximately 80% of metastases originate from carcinomas of breast, prostate, kidney, lung and the gastrointestinal tract.

With regard to fine needle aspiration cytology (FNAC) of bone lesions, the most important diagnostic use of cytology is when a single metastatic deposit is the presenting sign of a clinically silent tumour. According to Shih et al. [98] the kidney, lungs, liver, prostate and thyroid gland were the most common sources of solitary bone metastasis, while in a study by Katagiri et al. [99] the most common primary sites were the lungs, prostate, breasts and liver. Malignant melanoma is another not uncommon metastatic tumour in adults.

In paediatric patients, the most common neoplasms to give rise to bone metastases are rhabdomyosarcoma, neuroblastoma and clear-cell carcinoma of the kidney. Neuroblastoma typically metastatize to jaws, orbit and the metaphyses of the long bones. A solitary bone metastasis of neuroblastoma is not uncommonly diagnosed before the clinically occult primary tumour is found.

Radiology

Bone metastases are lytic or sclerotic. Lytic metastases are more common from breast, renal cell and lung carcinoma, while sclerotic metastases are commonly secondary to carcinoma of the prostate and the gastrointestinal canal. However, this does not always apply. Plain radiography is often the first diagnostic method used. Lytic metastases destroying the cortical bone are relatively easy to see, while central metastases within the bone marrow are impossible to diagnose by radiography. Sclerotic metastases are easier to see with plain radiography.

Bone scintigraphy is a common method to diagnose metastases, lytic as well as sclerotic. This is an efficient method because osteoblasts around the destruction are active, trying to repair the lesion and the radioactivity of the bone-seeking agents reflects the osteoblastic activity. However, bone scans may be negative when the lytic activity dominates and there is very little osteoblastic activity.

Unfortunately, there are many sources of false-positive bone scans in the search for metastatic deposits. Osteophytes on vertebral bodies, degenerative changes in connection with joints and sequelae after trauma such as fractures or infections may cause multiple active spots, simulating metastases. A combined evaluation of radiography and bone scintigraphy is mandatory in doubtful cases.

In recent years, MRI has proved to be a more efficient method to diagnose bone marrow metastases than radiography and bone scintigraphy, especially in the spine and long tubular bones. A total-body MRI with different sequences can be performed in the coronal plane of the body to efficiently and relatively rapidly reveal bone marrow lesions.

Recent developments of the CT technique have made it possible to examine the skeleton by whole-body CT. It is, however, difficult to diagnose lytic metastases in patients with general or local osteoporosis. The development of

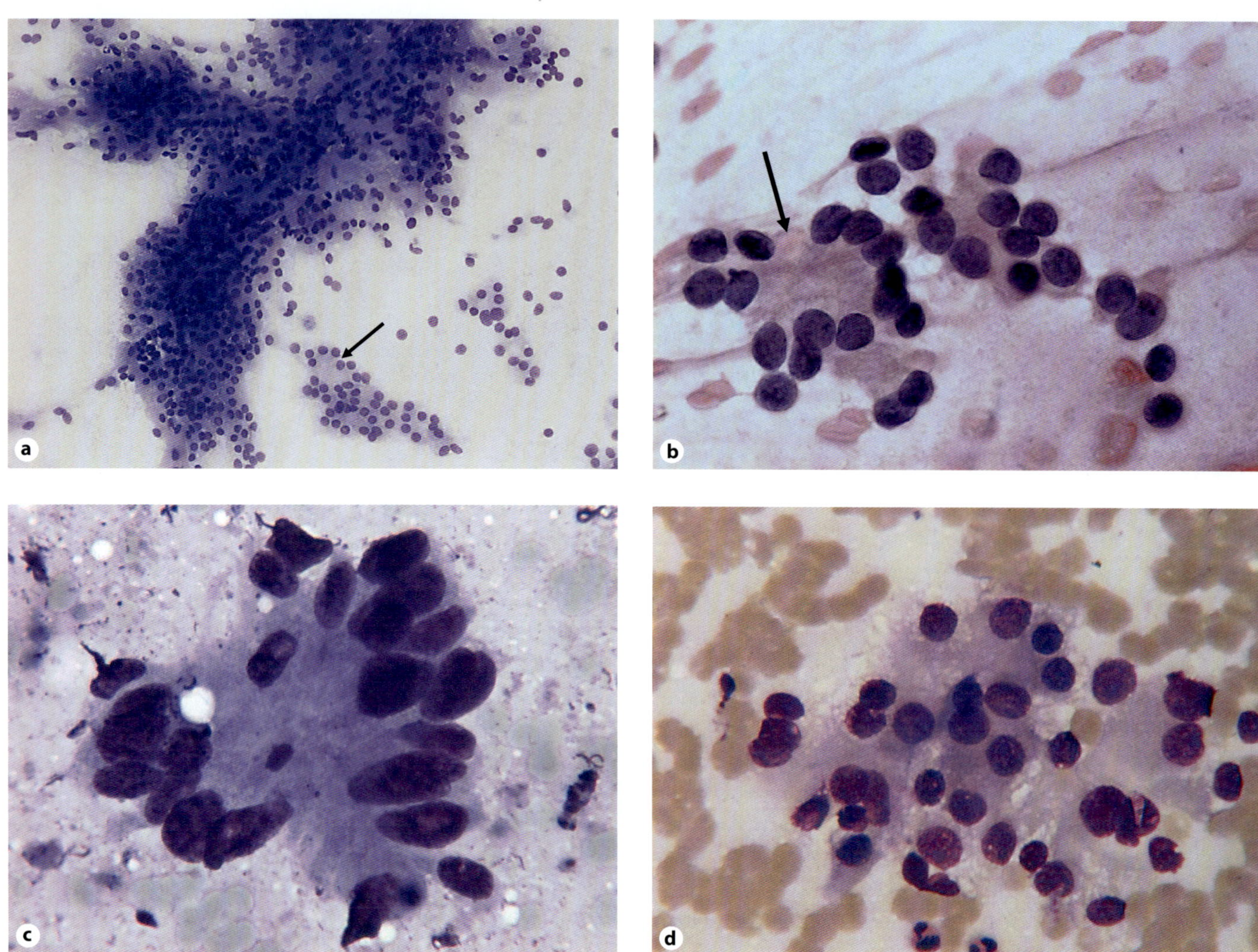

Fig. 77. Three examples of metastatic lesions with unknown primaries at needling in which it is possible to suggest the primary tumour. **a**, **b** Follicular thyroid carcinoma. Clusters of rather uniform, slightly atypical rounded tumour cells with follicular-like arrangement (arrows). MGG, low magnification (**a**). HE, medium magnification (**b**). **c** Colorectal carcinoma. Gland-like structure with atypical cylindrical cells. MGG, high magnification. **d** Renal carcinoma. A group of cytoplasm-rich cells with vacuolated cytoplasm and rounded nuclei. MGG, medium magnification.

PET-CT, a combination of radionuclear tests with CT is a very good diagnostic alternative, but the cost of such examinations are quite high.

Cytodiagnosis

The presence of gland-like structures is an important cytological feature in many bone metastases of carcinoma, but the main pattern of both poorly differentiated carcinoma and of melanoma is a mixture of single cells and loosely coherent cell clusters or groups of cells. The most important diagnostic use of FNAC is in cases in which a solitary destructive bone lesion is the first sign of a primary tumour elsewhere. In such cases, the cytopathologist should endeavour to identify or suggest the site of the primary tumour on the basis of the cytomorphology (fig. 77).

As mentioned, the commonest sites in adult patients are the kidneys, lungs, breasts, thyroid gland and colon. The cytological features of all these carcinomas are thoroughly described in current textbooks, as are common metastatic tumours in paediatric patients, neuroblastoma and rhabdomyosarcoma. It is important to apply adjunctive techniques, especially immunocytochemistry, in selected cases to accurately determine the primary site (fig. 78).

A number of useful antibodies are suggested in table 10.

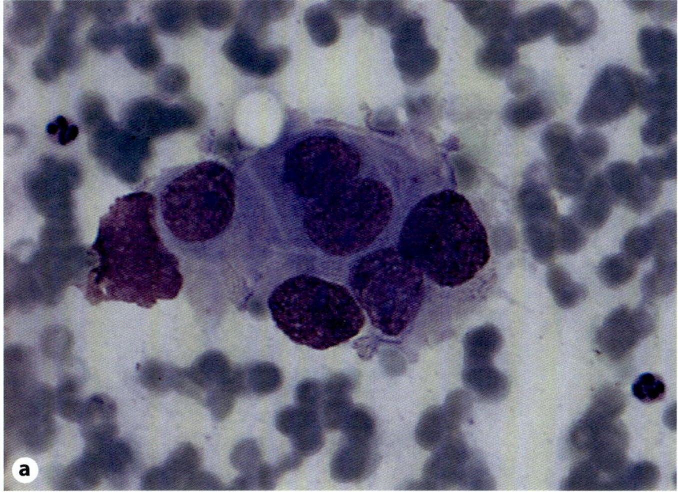
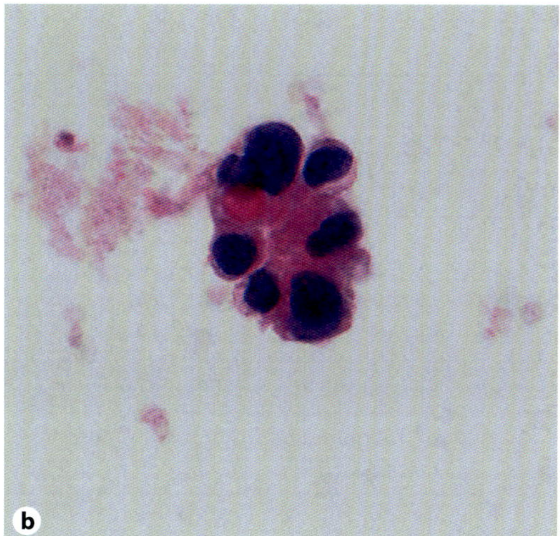
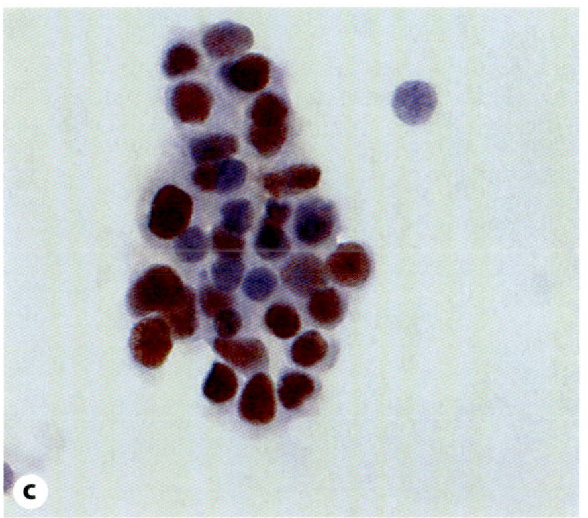
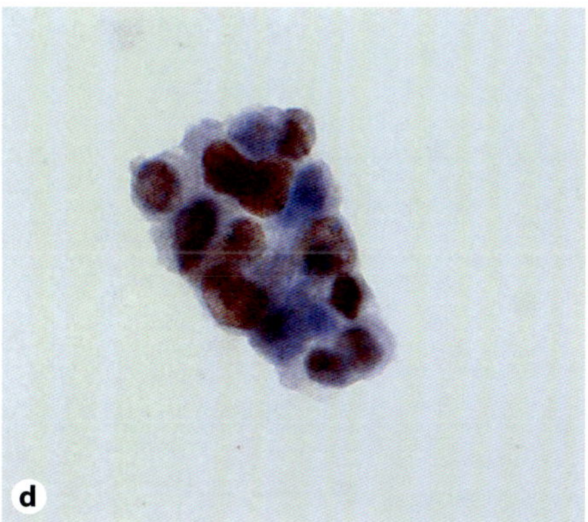

Fig. 78. The diagnostic use of immunocytochemistry is illustrated in this case of a metastatic breast carcinoma. **a**, **b** Adenocarcinoma with moderately atypical cells. MGG, high magnification (**a**). ThinPrep preparation, HE, medium magnification (**b**). **c** Oestrogen-receptor positive tumour cells. ThinPrep preparation, immunoperoxidase, medium magnification. **d** Progesterone-receptor positive tumour cells. ThinPrep preparation, immunoperoxidase, medium magnification.

Diagnostic Problems

There are a number of differential diagnostic problems in diagnosing metastatic bone disease.

Osteoblasts, especially when clustered, might look like mucin-producing carcinoma cells when the cytoplasmic 'Hof' is prominent.

Bone marrow cells, poorly preserved or smudged by smearing, can be mistaken for carcinoma cells especially when they are clumped. All 3 cell lines can be difficult to identify. Megakaryocytes can be mistaken for large tumour cells.

Poorly differentiated and pleomorphic plasmocytoma can be misinterpreted as anaplastic large-cell carcinoma, especially when the smearing results in clumping of cells resembling groups of epithelial cells.

As stated earlier, aspirates from chondrosarcoma and from chordoma may be misinterpreted as metastases from mucinous or clear-cell carcinoma when only wet-fixed material is available and the characteristic background matrix is weakly stained.

Case Report 6

The patient was a middle-aged male who had experienced pain in the left thorax for some time. There was no palpable tumour.

The radiological examination was a CT of the chest with the patient in prone position (fig. 79). There was destruction of the medial part of a left-sided rib close to the costovertebral joint (Th6), and a soft tissue extension of the lesion was also seen. In the figure, note that the needle was inserted from the back towards the lesion. The finding was non-specific and did not indicate the nature of the lesion.

Table 10. Antibodies suggested to apply in the type diagnosis of bone metastases.

Primary site/tumour	Antibody	Notes
Kidney	CK8/18, CK7/20, CD10	CK8/18+, CD10+, CK7/20–
Lung		
Squamous carcinoma	CK5/6, CK7	CK5/6+, CK7+/–
Adenocarcinoma	Ck7/20, TTF-1	Ck7+, TTF-1+, CK20–
Small-cell carcinoma	CK7/20, TTF-1	Ck7/20–, TTF-1+
Breast	CK7/20, ER, PR	CK7+, CK20–
Thyroid	thyreoglobulin, calcitonin, TTF-1	
Colon	CK7/20	CK20+, CK7–
Prostate	CK8/18, CK7/20, PSA	CK8/18+, CK7/20–
Melanoma	S-100, HMB45, MelanA	
Rhabdomyosarcoma	desmin, Myo-D1 (or Myogenin)	
Neuroblastoma	NSE, chromogranin	

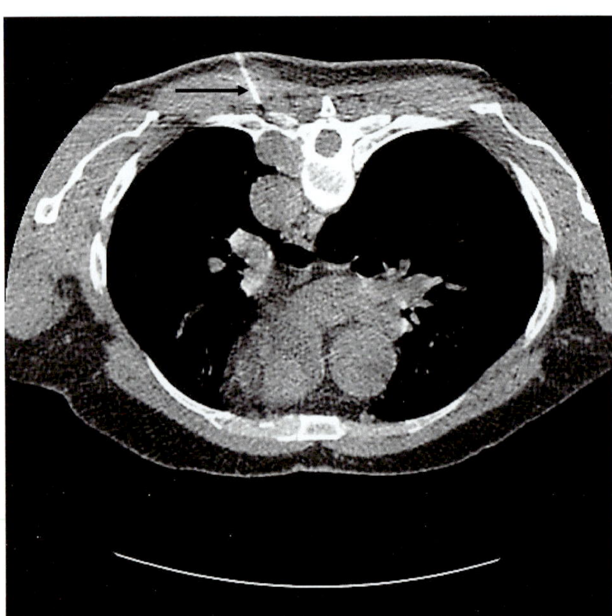

Fig. 79. Radiological features. CT examination of the chest with the patient in a prone position. There is a destruction of the medial part of a left-sided rib close to the costovertebral joint (Th6). There is a soft tissue extension of the lesion. Note the needle inserted from the back towards the lesion (arrow). The finding is non-specific and does not indicate the nature of the lesion.

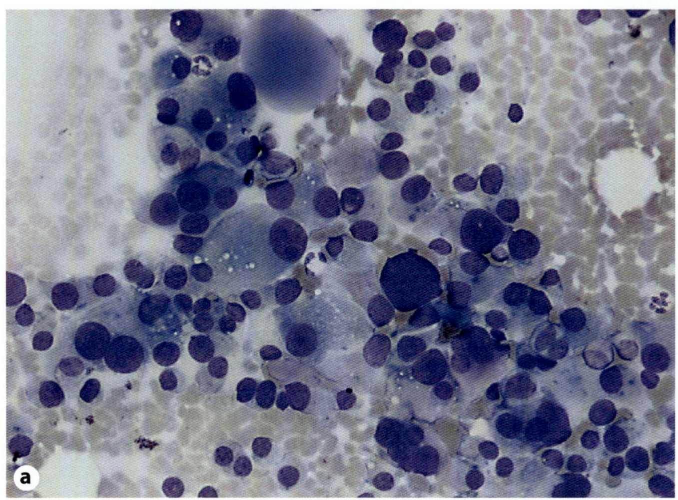

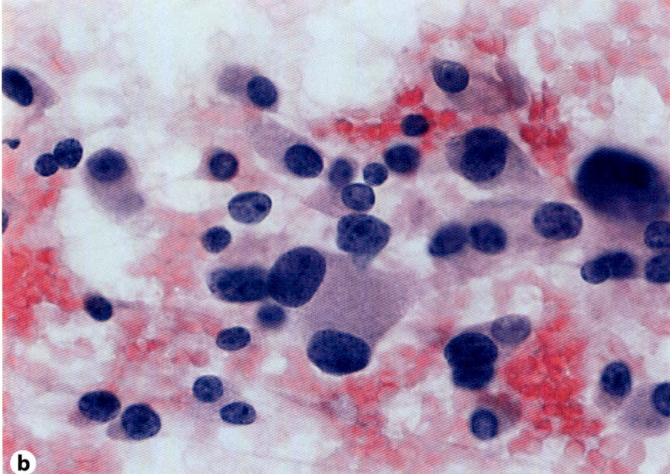

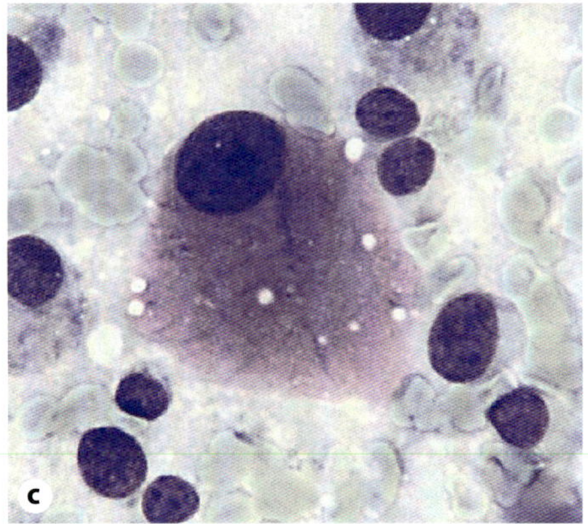

Fig. 80. **a** Rich cell yield. Predominantly dispersed malignant cells displaying a marked variation in size and shape. Multinucleated tumour cells are present. MGG, low magnification. **b**, **c** The larger tumour cells have an abundant cytoplasm and eccentric nuclei. The cell shown in **c** displays a fine, red cytoplasmic granulation. HE, high magnification (**b**). MGG, high magnification (**c**).

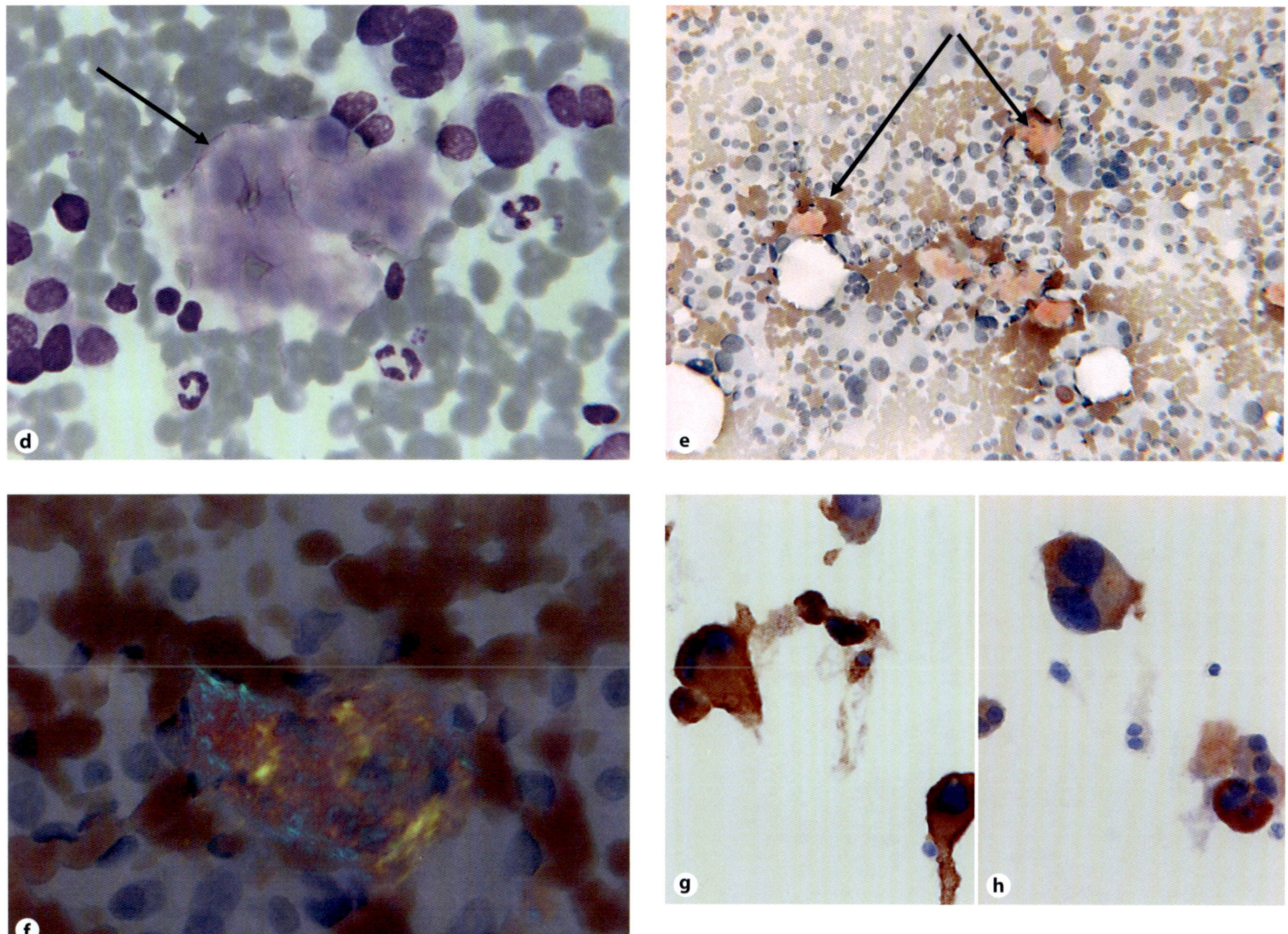

Fig. 80. **d** Clumps of a hyaline blue-grey material are present between the tumour cells (arrow). MGG, high magnification. **e** Small amyloid deposits staining reddish. Kongo, medium magnification. **f** The amyloid deposits appear greenish in polarized light. Medium magnification. **g** Strong cytoplasmic staining with calcitonin. ThinPrep preparation, immunoperoxidase, high magnification. **h** Strong cytoplasmic staining with chromogranin A. ThinPrep preparation, high magnification.

CT-guided aspiration was performed by the radiologist.

From the aspiration, there was a rich cellular yield (fig. 80a; MGG, low magnification). As can be seen from the figure, dispersed malignant cells displaying a marked variation in size and shape predominate. Multinucleated tumour giant cells are present.

Fig. 80b (HE and 80c MGG, high magnification). The larger tumour cells have abundant cytoplasm and eccentric nuclei. A fine red cytoplasmic granulation is evident in figure 80c (MGG, high magnification). Clumps of hyaline blue/grey material are seen between the tumour cells (fig. 80d; MGG, high magnification).

The microscopic findings clearly indicated that the smears originated from a malignant tumour. Although the large tumour cells could suggest an osteosarcoma, the marked variation in size and the lack of strands of red/violet stained osteoid were features against this diagnosis. Myxoid or hyaline matrix, typically present in high-grade chondrosarcoma, was not seen. The favoured diagnosis was of a metastatic deposit and the large tumour cells with red cytoplasmic granulation and eccentric nuclei, together with the clumps of blue-grey hyaline material, suggested a metastasis from a medullary carcinoma of the thyroid gland.

One smear was destained and restained showing typically red-stained amyloid that appeared greenish in polarized light (fig. 80e; Kongo stain, medium magnification; fig. 80f; medium magnification).

In figure 80 (ThinPrep immunoperoxidase, high magnification), the tumour cells show strong cytoplasmic staining with calcitonin (fig. 80g) and chromogranin A (fig. 80h).

The final cytological diagnosis was metastasis from a medullary carcinoma of the thyroid. Further investigations confirmed a medullary carcinoma of the thyroid.

Comments

The radiological investigation showed a non-specific destruction with a soft tissue extension with no typical signs of osteo- or chondrosarcoma. The clues to the cytological diagnosis were the large cytoplasm-rich cells with red granulation and eccentric nuclei, and the intercellular hyaline clumps not typical for osteoid or cartilaginous matrix.

Chapter 14

Fine Needle Aspiration as the First Diagnostic Modality for Spinal and Sacral Lesions

Primary bone tumours/lesions and metastatic bone disease are not uncommon in the spine and sacrum. When bone metastasis is the first manifestation of a malignant tumour, the spine is the site of the lesion in about 80% of cases. Fine needle aspiration cytology (FNAC) is preferable to open biopsy or core needle biopsy as the primary modality to reach a morphological diagnosis in these sites.

A correctly guided FNA, in most cases ambulatory, has a high diagnostic accuracy. The diagnostic efficacy of FNAC in evaluating bone tumours/lesions in the vertebrae and sacrum has been documented in several series [8, 18, 100, 101]. In our experience, FNAC differentiates primary benign and malignant bone tumours from metastatic deposits with a high degree of diagnostic accuracy and furthermore pinpoints the site of the primary tumour in most cases. The radiographic findings in these sites are often not specific enough to suggest a histotype. Many different lesions including some benign ones appear radiographically lytic/destructive, for example conventional giant-cell tumours in the sacrum, osteoblastoma in the vertebral bodies and plasmocytoma and metastasis in the sacrum. In these sites, FNAC is a most valuable diagnostic complement to the radiographic findings.

The following case reports, taken from our files, demonstrate the diagnostic power of guided aspiration in lesions of the vertebrae and sacrum.

Case Report 7

The patient was a middle-aged male complaining of low back pain.

The radiological examination showed a destructive lesion in the ninth thoracic vertebra to the left with penetration into the spinal canal (fig. 81). The finding was non-specific and did not indicate the nature of the lesion.

FNA was performed by the radiologist.

Figure 82a (MGG, low magnification) shows a haemorrhagic aspirate with several large multinucleated, osteoclast-like cells. In figure 82b (MGG) and 82c (HE, medium magnification) dispersed or clustered mononuclear cells with rather uniform rounded, at times eccentric, nuclei are visible.

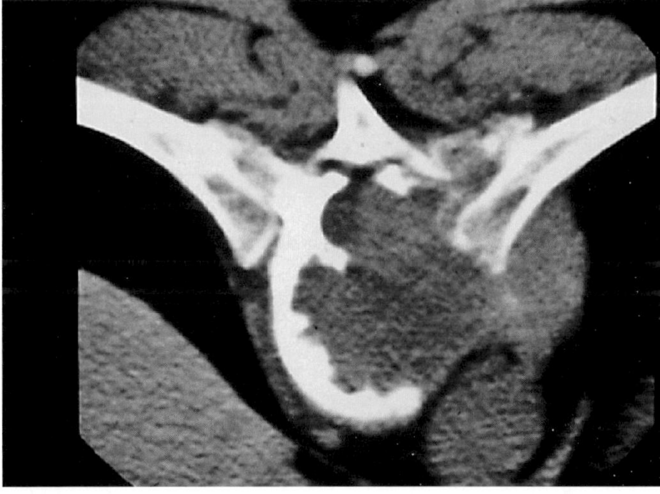

Fig. 81. Radiological features. CT examination of the spine with the patient in a prone position. There is a destructive lesion in the right aspect of the ninth thoracal vertebra with penetration into the spinal canal and with a paravertebral extension. The finding is non-specific and does not indicate the nature of the lesion.

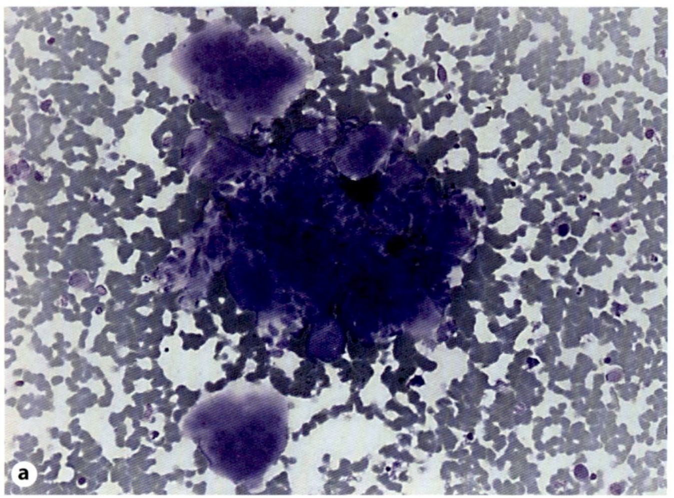

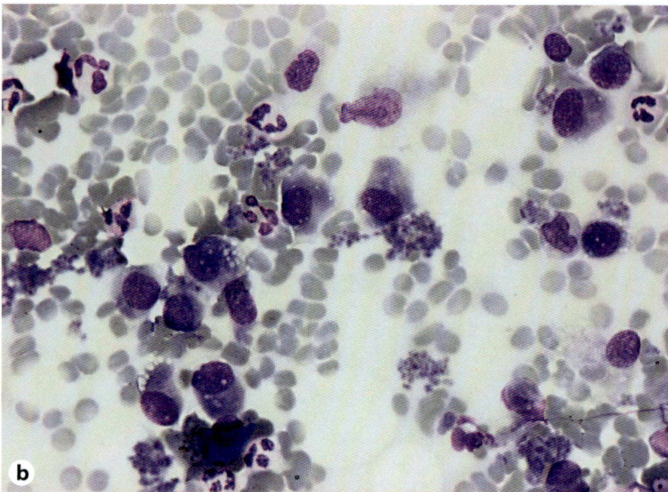

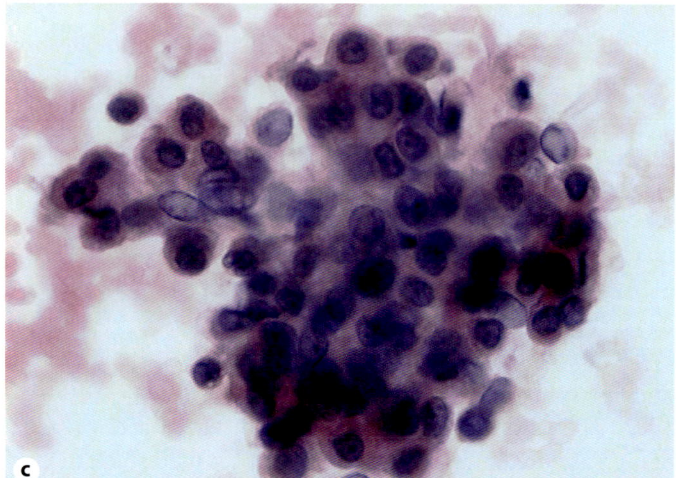

Fig. 82. **a** Haemorrhagic aspirate with several large multinucleated osteoclast-like cells. MGG, low magnification. **b**, **c**. Dispersed or clustered mononuclear cells with rather uniform rounded, at times eccentric nuclei. **b** MGG, medium magnification. **c**. HE, medium magnification.

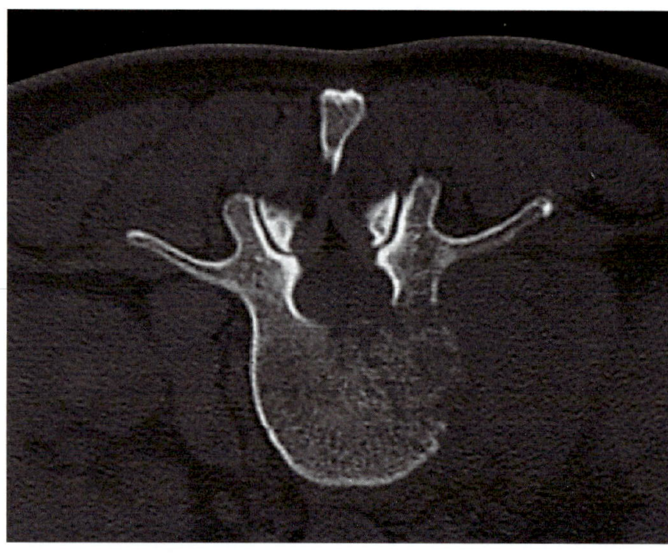

Fig. 83. Radiological features. CT of the spine in prone position. Bone destruction of the right aspect of the L2 vertebra. The destruction is of permeative nature also with a soft tissue component in the right psoas muscle. The destruction is non-specific and does not indicate the nature of the lesion.

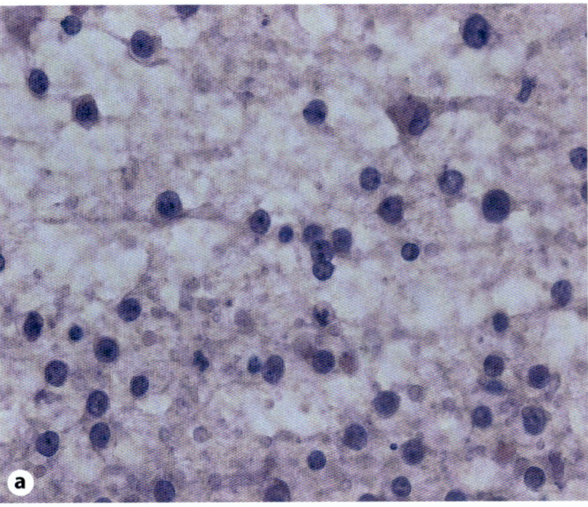

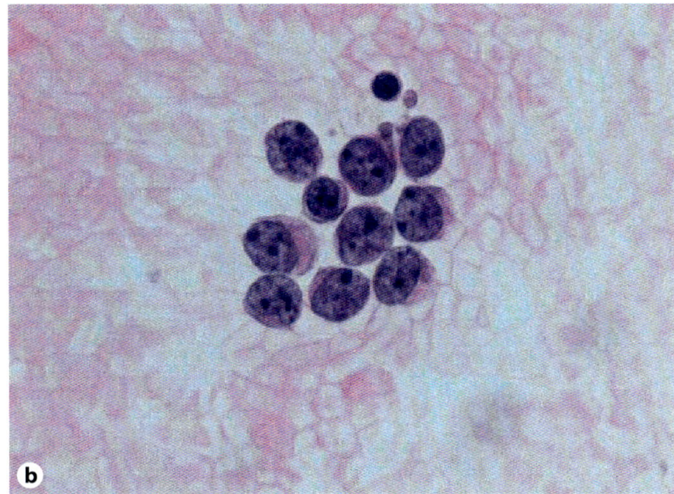

Fig. 84. a Dispersed tumour cells with scanty cytoplasm and rounded nuclei present on a haemorrhagic back ground. HE, medium magnification. **b** At high magnification the tumour cells have a characteristic appearance of centroblasts: a narrow cytoplasmic brim around rounded nuclei with distinct nucleoli, often alongside the nuclear membrane. HE, high magnification.

The cytology excluded a malignant tumour. The double cell population with osteoclast-like cells and mononuclear cells suggested a giant-cell tumour or osteoblastoma. The cytologist reported the lesion as a 'benign primary bone tumour with multiple osteoclast-like cells'.

The subsequent operative specimen was histologically diagnosed as a giant-cell tumour.

Case Report 8

The patient was a middle-aged female, who was referred for lower back pain with the accompanying notes: 'Destruction right part of the L2 vertebra. Primary unknown'.

The radiological examination was a CT of the spine with the patient in a prone position (fig. 83). It showed bone destruction of the right aspect of the L2 vertebra. The destruction was of permeative nature and associated with a soft tissue component in the right psoas muscle. The destruction is non-specific and does not indicate the nature of the lesion.

FNA was performed by the radiologist.

Figure 84a (HE Medium magnification) shows dispersed tumour cells with scanty cytoplasm and rounded nuclei present on a haemorrhagic background. At high magnification (Fig. 84b; HE) the tumour cells have the characteristic appearance of centroblasts: a small cytoplasmic brim around rounded nuclei with distinct nucleoli, often alongside the nuclear membrane.

The tumour cells had the appearances of centroblasts and an aggressive non-Hodgkin lymphoma was suspected. Part of the aspirate was submitted to flow cytometric phenotyping, which showed lambda monoclonal B-cells.

The cytological diagnosis was diffuse large-cell B-cell lymphoma.

Case Report 9

The patient was an elderly female complaining of low back pain who was referred for investigation with the following notes: 'Metastatic tumour in the L5 vertebra. Primary unknown, however breast carcinoma 13 years ago'.

The radiological examination was a T1-W axial MRI sequence of the lumbar spine (fig. 85). Extensive low-signal tumour growth in the vertebral body and the posterior elements of L5.

FNA was performed by the radiologist.

Figures 86a (MGG, medium magnification) and 86b (HE, high magnification) show groups of tumour cells with moderately atypical nuclei. Vaguely outlined glandlike structures are visible (arrow in the figure).

The preliminary cytological diagnosis was metastatic adenocarcinoma, probably from the breast carcinoma.

Figures 86c (ThinPrep Immunoperoxidase oestrogen receptor, high magnification) and 86d (ThinPrep immunoperoxidase progesterone receptor, high magnification) show focal positive nuclear staining.

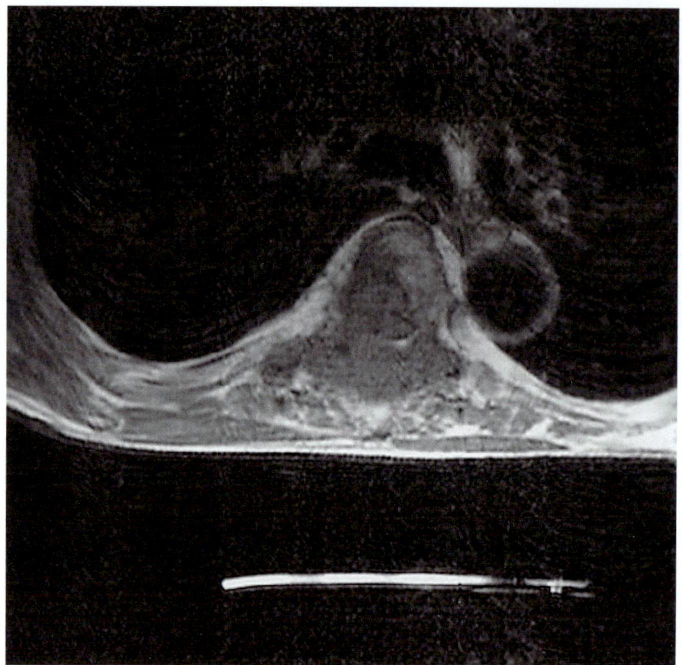

Fig. 85. Radiological features. T1-weighted axial MRI sequence of the lumbar spine. Extensive low-signal tumour growth in the vertebral body and posterior elements of L5.

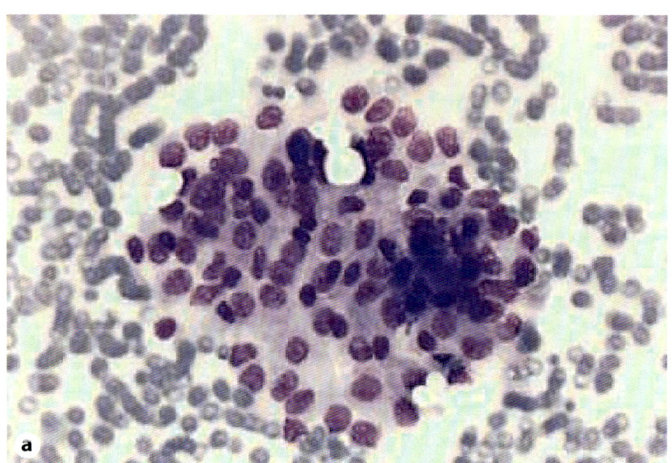

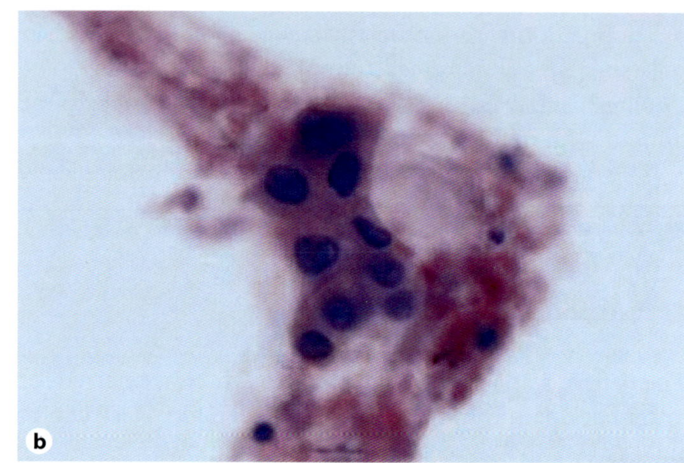

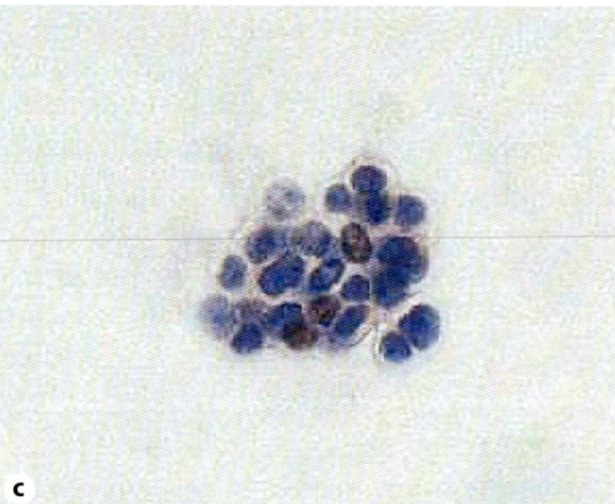

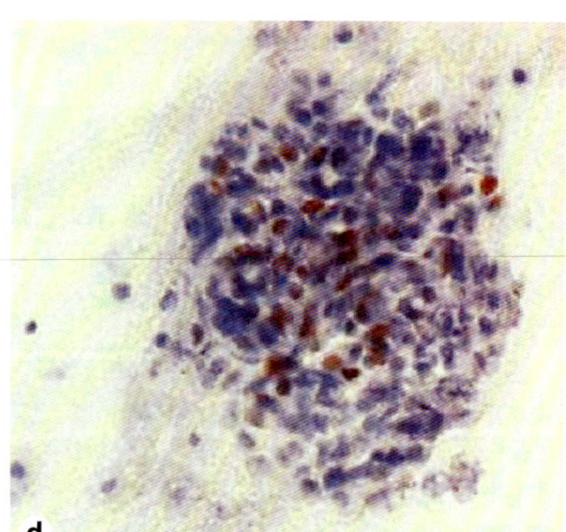

Fig. 86. a, **b** Groups of tumour cells with moderately atypical nuclei. Faintly outlined glandlike structures (arrow). MGG, medium magnification (**a**). HE, high magnification (**b**). **c** Focal positive nuclear staining with oestrogen receptor. ThinPrep preparation, immunoperoxidase, high magnification. **d** Focal positive nuclear staining with progesterone receptor. ThinPrep preparation, immunoperoxidase, medium magnification.

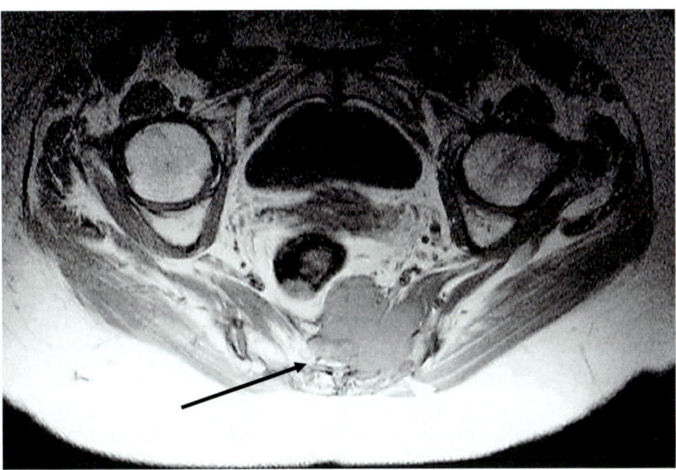

Fig. 87. Radiological features. T1-weighted axial MRI section of the pelvis. There is a destruction of the left side of sacrum, with soft tissue extension anteriorly (arrow).

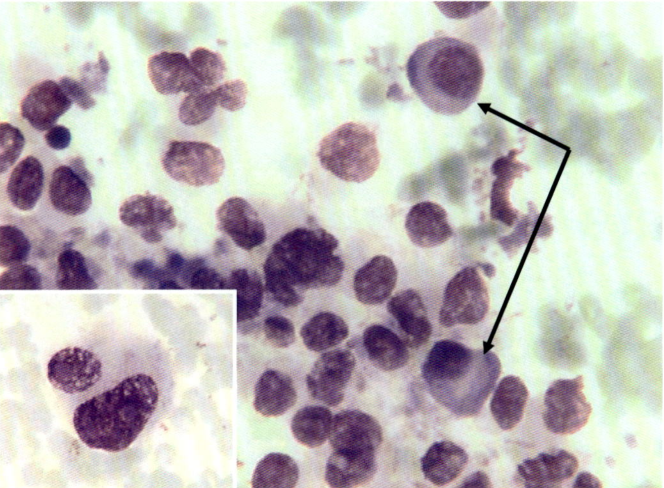

Fig. 88. Dispersed tumour cells with irregular, often striped nuclei. Among them, 2 preserved moderately atypical plasma cells are seen (arrows). MGG, medium magnification. Inset shows a highly atypical binucleated plasma cell. MGG, high magnification.

The final cytological diagnosis was metastasis of breast carcinoma to L5 vertebra.

Case Report 10

The patient was an elderly female. She had previously undergone surgery for poorly differentiated squamous cell carcinoma of the vulva with lympnode metastasis to the right groin. A lesion in the sacrum was discovered 8 months after the primary treatment.

FNA was performed by the radiologist.

The radiological examination was aT1-weighted axial section of the pelvis (fig. 87). There was destruction of the left side of the sacrum, with soft tissue extension anteriorly (arrow in the figure).

Figure 88 (MGG, medium magnification) shows dispersed tumour cells with irregular, often striped nuclei. Among them, 2 well preserved moderately atypical plasmacells are seen (arrows). The inset image (MGG, high magnification) shows a highly atypical binucleated plasma cell.

Further evaluation with immunohistochemistry on a cell block preparation from the aspirate revealed a kappa monoclonal cellular population. Cytokeratins were negative.

The cytological diagnosis was solitary plasmacytoma. There was no sign of carcinoma metastasis.

Comments

The radiologic investigations in all 4 cases diagnosed destructive lesions, some of them with a soft tissue extension, but could not specifically suggest a diagnosis.

The cases illustrate the value of guided aspirations performed by radiologists trained in the aspiration technique. Surgical or core needle biopsy was not performed in any of the cases before the definitive treatment

Summary and Conclusions

FNAC used in the primary work-up of bone tumours/lesions is an effective and accurate diagnostic modality. When the diagnosis is based on the combined evaluation of clinical data, radiographic findings and cytological features, open biopsy before definitive treatment is not necessary in most cases. The optimal use of FNA is reached when patients are referred to a multidisciplinary centre with a close cooperation between the cytopathologist, radiologist and orthopaedic surgeon.

Outside such centres, it is mandatory for the cytopathologist to collect all available clinical and radiographic information and to base the definitive diagnosis on the combined evaluation of clinical, radiographic and cytological data: the clinical, radiological, cytological approach.

References

1 Stormby N, Åkerman M: Cytodiagnosis of bone lesions by means of fine-needle aspiration. Acta Cytol 1973;17:166–172.
2 Dorfman H, Czerniak B: Bone Tumors. St Louis, Mosby, 1997.
3 Dahlin DC, Unni KK: Bone Tumors. General aspects and data on 8,542 cases, ed 4. Springfield, Charles C Thomas, 1986.
4 Pramesh CS, Deshpande MS, Pardiwala DN, Agarwal MG, Puri A: Core needle biopsy for bone tumours. Eur J Surg Oncol 2001;27:668–671.
5 Jelinek JS, Murphey MD, Welker JA, Henshaw RM, Kransdorf MJ, Shmookler BM, Malawer MM: Diagnosis of primary bone tumors with image-guided percutaneous biopsy: experience with 110 tumors. Radiology 2002;223:731–737.
6 Ossakov J, Flusser G, Kollender Y, Merimsky O, Lifschitz-Mercer B, Meller I: Computed tomography-guided core needle biopsy for bone and soft tissue tumors. Isr Med Assoc J 2003;5:28–30.
7 Viellard MH, Boutry N, Chastanet P, Duquesnoy B, Cotton A, Cortet B: Contribution of percutaneous biopsy in the definitive diagnosis in patients with suspected bone tumor. Joint Bone Spine 2005;72:53–60.
8 Coley BL, Sharp GS, Ellis EB: Diagnosis of bone tumors by aspiration. Am J Surg 1931;13:214–224.
9 Åkerman M, Berg NO, Persson B: Fine needle aspiration biopsy in the evaluation of tumor-like lesions of bone. Acta Orthop Scand 1976;47: 129–136.
10 Palombini L, Marino D, Vetrani A, Fulciniti F: Fine-needle aspiration biopsy on primary malignant and metastatic bone tumors. Appl Pathol 1983;1:76–81.
11 Layfield L, Armstrong K, Zaleski S, Eckhardt J: Diagnostic accuracy and clinical utility of fine-needle aspiration cytology in the diagnosis of clinically primary bone tumors. Diagn Cytopathol 1993;9:168–173.
12 Kreicsbergs A, Bauer HCF; Brosjö O, Linsholm J, Skoog L, Söderlund V: Cytological diagnosis of bone tumours. J Bone Joint Surg (B) 1996;78-B: 258–263.
13 Bommer KK, Ramzay I, Mody D: Fine-needle aspiration in the diagnosis and management of bone lesions: a study of 450 cases. Cancer 1997; 81:148–156.
14 Kabukcuoglu F, Kabukcuoglu Y, Kuzgun U, Evren I: Fine needle aspiration of malignant bone lesions. Acta Cytol 1998;42:875–882.
15 Åkerman M, Domanski HA: Fine needle aspiration (FNA) of bone tumours: with special emphasis on definitive treatment of primary malignant bone tumours based on FNA. Curr Diagn Pathol 1998;5:82–92.
16 Jorda M, Rey L, Hanly A, Ganjei-Azar P: Fine-needle aspiration cytology of bone. Accuracy and pitfalls of cytodiagnosis. Cancer 2000;90:47–54.
17 Agarwal AS, Agarwal T, Agarwal IR, Agarwal PK, Jain UK: Fine needle aspiration of bone tumors. Cancer Detect Prev 2000;24:602–609.
18 Söderlund V, Skoog L, Kreicbergs A: Combined radiology and cytology in the diagnosis of bone lesions: a retrospective study of 370 cases. Acta Orthop Scand 2004;75:492–499.
19 Ahlström KH, Åström KG: CT-guided bone biopsy performed by means of a coaxial biopsy system with an eccentric drill. Radiology 1993;188:549–552.
20 Bauer HCF, Kreicberga A, Silfversvärd C: DNA analysis in the differential diagnosis of osteosarcoma. Cancer 1988;61:2532–2540.
21 Kreicbergs A, Zetterberg A, Söderberg G: The prognostic significance of nuclear DNA content in chondrosarcoma. Anal Quant Cytol 1980;2: 272–279.
22 Kusuzaki K, Murata H, Takeshita H, Hirata M, Haschiguchi S, Nakamura S, Ashihara T, Hirasawa Y: Usefulness of cytofluorometric DNA ploidy analysis in distinguishing benign cartilaginous tumours from chondrosarcoma. Mod Pathol 1999;12:863–872.
23 Åkerman M, Dreinhöfer K, Rydholm A, Willén H, Mertens F, Mitelman F, Mandahl N: Cytogenetic studies on fine-needle aspiration samples from osteosarcoma and Ewing's sarcoma. Diagn Cytopathol 1996;15:17–22.
24 Udayakumar AM, Sundareshan TS, Goud TM, Devi MG, Biswas S, Appaji L, Aruakumari BS, Rajan KR, Prabhakaren PS: Cytogentic characterization of Ewing's tumors using fine needle aspiration samples: a 10-year experience and review of the literature. Cancer Genet Cytogenet 2001;127:42–48.
25 Fröstad B: Fine Needle Aspiration Cytology in the Diagnosis and Management of Childhood Small Round Cell Tumours; thesis, Stockholm, 2000.
26 Söderlund V: Combined Radiology and Cytology in the Diagnosis of Bone Lesions; thesis, Stockholm, 2002.
27 McLaughlin RE, Miller WR, Miller CW: Quadriparesis after needle aspiration of the cervical spine. J Bone Joint Surg 1976;58:1167–1168.
28 Rööser B, Herrlin K, Rydholm A, Åkerman M: Pseudomalignant myositis ossificans: clinical, radiologic, and cytologic diagnosis in 5 cases. Acta Orthop Scand 1989;60:457–460.
29 Wakely PE Jr, Almeida M, Frable WJ: Fine-needle aspiration biopsy cytology of myositis ossificans. Mod Pathol 1994;7:23–25.
30 Fletcher CDM, Unni KK, Mertens F: Pathology and genetics: tumours of soft tissue and bone. World Health Organization classification of tumours. Lyon, IARC Press, 2002.
31 Waalas L, Kindblom LG: Light and electron microscopic examination of fine-needle aspirates in the preoperative diagnosis of osteogenic tumors: a study of 21 osteosarcomas and two osteoblastomas. Diagn Cytopathol 1990;6: 27–38.
32 Rhode MG, Lucas DR, Krueger CH, Pu RT: Fine-needle aspiration of spinal osteoblastoma in a patient with lymfangiomatosis. Diagn Cytopathol 2006;34:295–297.
33 Bertoni F, Bacchini P, Donati D, Martini A, Picci P, Campamacci M: Osteoblastoma-like osteosarcoma: the Rizzoli Institute experience. Mod Pathol 1993;6:707–716.
34 White WA, Fanning CV, Ayala AG, Raymond KA, Carrasco HC, Murray JA: Osteosarcoma and the role of fine-needle aspiration: a study of 51 cases. Cancer 1988;62:1238–1246.

35 Bhatia A, Ashokraj G: Cytological diversity of osteosarcoma. Indian J Cancer 1992;29:56–60.
36 Dodd LG, Scully SP, Cothran RL, Harrelson JM: Utility of fine-needle aspiration in the diagnosis of primary osteosarcoma. Diagn Cytopathol 2002;27:350–353.
37 Domanski HA, Åkerman M: Fine-needle aspiration of primary osteosarcoma: a cytological-histological study. Diagn Cytopathol 2005;32:269–275.
38 Klijanienko J, Caillaud J-M, Orbach D, Brisse H, Lagacé R, Sastre-Gareau X: Cyto-histological correlations in primary, recurent and metastatic bone and soft tissue osteosarcoma. Institut Curie´s experience. Diagn Cytopathol 2007;35: 270–275.
39 Serra M, Morini MC, Scotlandi K, Fisher LW, Zini N, Colombo MP, Campanacci M, Maraldi NM, Olivari S, Baldini N: Evaluation of osteonectin as a diagnostic marker of osteogenic bone tumors. Human Pathol 1992;23:1326–1331.
40 Fanburg JC, Rosenberg AE, Weaver DL, Laslie KO, Mann KG, Taatjes DJ, Tracy RP: Osteocalcin and osteonectin immunoreactivity in the diagnosis of osteosarcoma. Am J Clin Pathol 1997;108 464–473.
41 Park SH, Kim I: Small cell osteosarcoma of the ribs: immunohistochemical, and ultrastructural study with literature review. Ultrastruct Pathol 1999;23:133–140.
42 Waalas L, Kindblom L-G, Gunterberg B, Bergh P: Light and electron-microscopic examination of fine needle aspiration in the preoperative diagnosis of cartilaginous tumours. Diagn Cytopathol 1990;6:396–408.
43 Dhawan SB, Aggarwal R, Mohan H, Kumar S: Cytodiagnosis of enchondroma. Cytopathology 2003;14:157–159.
44 Fanning CV, Sneige NS, Carrasco CH, Ayala AG, Murray JA, Raymond AK: Fine needle aspiration cytology of chondroblastoma of bone. Cancer 1990;65:1847–1863.
45 Pohar-Marinsek Z, Us-Krasovec M, Lamovee J: Chondroblastoma in fine needle aspirates. Acta Cytol 1992;36:367–370.
46 Kilpatrick SE, Pike EJ, Geisinger KR, Ward WG: Chondroblastoma of bone: use of fine-needle aspiration biopsy and potential diagnostic pitfalls. Diagn Cytopathol 1997;16:65–71.
47 Bhatia A: Problems in the interpretation of bone tumours with fine needle aspiration (letter). Acta Cytol 1984;28:91–92.
48 Layfield LJ, Ferreiro JA: Fine-needle aspiration cytology of chondromyxoid fibroma: a case report. Diagn Cytopathol 1988;4:148–151.
49 Gupta S, Dev G, Marya S: Chondromyxoid fibroma: a fine-needle aspiration diagnosis. Diagn Cytopathol 1993;9:63–65.
50 Tunc M, Ekinci C: Chondrosarcoma diagnosed by fine needle aspiration cytology. Acta Cytol 1996; 40:283–288.
51 Lerma E, Tani E, Brosjö O, Bauer HC, Söderlund V, Skoog L: Diagnosis and grading of chondrosarcoma on FNA biopsy material. Diagn Cytopathol 2003;28:13–17.
52 Dodd LG: Fine needle aspiration of chondrosarcoma. Diagn Cytopathol 2006;34:413–418.
53 Bauer HC, Brosjö O, Kreicbergs A, Lindholm J: Low risk of recurrence of enchondroma and low-grade chondrosarcoma in extremities. Acta Orthop Scand 1995;66:283–288.
54 Dee S, Meneses N, Ostrowski ML, Horowitz M, Graf W: Pleomorphic ('dedifferentiated') chondrosarcoma: report of a case initially examined by fine needle aspiration biopsy. Acta Cytol 1991;35:467–471.
55 Rinas AC, Ward WG, Kilpatrick SE: Potential sampling error in fine needle aspiration biopsy of dedifferentiated chondrosarcoma: a report of 4 cases. Acta Cytol 2005;49:554–559.
56 Dhener LP: Primitive neuroectodermal tumor and Ewing's sarcoma. Am J Surg Pathol 1993;17:1–13.
57 Delattre O, Zucman J, Melot T, Garau XS, Zucker JM, Lenoir GM, Ambros PF, Sheer D, Turc-Carel C, Triche TJ: The Ewing family of tumours: a subgroup of small-roundcell tumors defined by specific chimeric transcripts. N Engl Med J 1994;331:294–299.
58 Llombart-Bosch A, Navarro S: Immunohistochemical detection of EWS and FLI-1 proteins in Ewing sarcoma and primitive neuroectodermal tumors: comparative analysis with CD99 (MIC-2) expression. Appl Immunohistochem Mol Morphol 2001;9:255–260.
59 Folpe AL, Hill CE, Parham DM, O'Shea PA, Weiss SW: Immunohistochemical detection of FLI-1 protein expression: a study of 132 round cell tumors with emphasis on CD99-positive mimics of Ewing's sarcoma/primitive neuroectodermal tumor. Am J Surg Pathol 2000;24:1657–1662.
60 Angervall L, Enzinger FM: Extraskeletal neoplasm resembling Ewing's sarcoma. Cancer 1975;36:240–251.
61 Akhtar M, Ali MA, Sabbah R: Aspiration cytology of Ewing's sarcoma. Light and electron microscopic correlations. Cancer 1985;56:2051–2060.
62 Dahl I, Åkerman M, Angervall L: Ewing's sarcoma of bone. A correlative cytological and histological study of 14 cases. Acta Pathol Microbiol Immunol Scand (A) 1986;94:363–369.
63 Silverman JS, Berns LA, Holbrook CT, Neill JS, Joshi VV: Fine needle aspiration cytology of primitive neuroectodermal tumors: a report of these cases. Acta Cytol 1992;36:541–550.
64 Mondal A, Misra DK: Ewing´s sarcoma of bone: a study of 71 cases by fine needle aspiration cytology. J Indian Med Assoc 1996;94:135–137.
65 Renshaw AA, Parez-Atayde AR, Fletcher JA, Granter SR: Cytology of typical and atypical Ewing's sarcoma/PNET. Am J Surg Pathol 1996;106:620–624.
66 Guiter GE, Gamboni MM, Zakowski MF: The cytology of extraskeletal Ewing sarcoma. Cancer 1999;87:141–148.
67 Sahu K, Pai RR, Khadikar UN: Fine needle aspiration cytology of the Ewing's sarcoma family of tumors. Acta Cytol 2000;332–336.
68 Olsen SH, Thomas DG, Lucas DR: Cluster analysis of immunohistochemical profiles in synovial sarcoma, malignant peripheral nerve sheath tumor, and Ewing sarcoma. Mod Pathol 2006; 19:659–668.
69 Waalas L, KindblomL-G: Fine needle aspiration biopsy in the preoperative diagnosis of chordoma: a study of 17 cases with application of electron microscopy, histochemical and immunohistochemical examination. Human Pathol 1990;22:22–28.
70 Finley JL, Silverman JF, Dabbs DJ, West RI, Dickens A, Feldman PS, Frable WJ: Chordoma: diagnosis by fine-needle aspiration with histologic, immnuocytochemical, and ultrastructural confirmation. Diagn Cytopathol 1998;2: 330–337.
71 Crapanzano JP, Ali Sz, Ginsberg MS, Zakowski MF: Chordoma: a cytologic study with histologic and radiologic correlation. Cancer 2001;93:40–51.
72 Kay PA, Nasciemento AG, Unni KK, Salomao DR: Chordoma: cytomorphologic findings in 14 cases diagnosed by fine needle aspiration. Acta Cytol 2003;47:202–208.
73 Kumar MD, Misra K: Fine needle aspiration cytodiagnosis of subcutaneous sacrococcygeal myxopapillary ependymoma: a case report. Acta Cytol 1990;34:851–854.
74 Kulesza P, Tihan T, Ali SZ: Myxopapillary ependymoma: cytomorphologic characteristics and differential diagnosis. Diagn Cytopathol 2002;26:247–250.
75 Layfield LJ: Cytologic differential diagnosis of myxoid and mucinous neoplasms of the sacrum and parasacral soft tissues. Diagn Cytopathol 2003;28:264–271.
76 Sneige N, Ayala GA, Carrasco CH, Murray J, Raymond AK: Giant cell tumor of bone: a cytologic study of 24 cases. Diagn Cytopathol 1985;1:111–117.
77 Vetrani A, Fulciniti F, Boschi R, Marino G, Zeppa P, Troncone G, Palombini L: Fine needle aspiration biopsy diagnosis of giant-cell tumor of bone. Acta Cytol 1990;34:863–867.
78 Yamamato T, Nagira K, Akisu T, Marui T, Hitora T, Kawamoto T, Yoshia S, Kurosaka M, Tsukamoto R: Fine-needle aspiration biopsy of solid aneurysmal bone cyst in the humerus. Diagn Cytopathol 2003;28:159–162.
79 Watson CW, Unger P, Kaneko M, Gabrilove JL: Fine needle aspiration of osteitis fibrosa cystica. Diagn Cytopathol 1985;1:157–160.
80 Gupta RK, Voss DM, McHutchinson AG, Hatfield PJ: Osteitis fibrosa cystica (brown tumor) in a patient with renal transplantation. Acta Cytol 1992;36:555–558.
81 Troncone G, Vetrani A, Boschi R: Il difetto fibroso metafisarion (DFM) in biopsia per ago sottile. Istocitopatologia 1988;10:113–118.
82 Logrono R, Kurtycs DF, Wojtowyes M, Inhorn S: Fine needle aspiration cytology of fibrous dysplasia: a case report. Acta Cytol 1998;42:1172–1176.
83 Czerniak B, Rojas-Corona RR, Dorfman HD: Morphologic diversity of long bone adamantinoma; the concept of differentiated (regressing) adamantinoma and its relationship to osteofibrous dysplasia. Cancer 1989;64:2319–2334.

84 Campanacci M, Giunti A, Bertoni F, Laus M, Gitelis S: Adamantinoma of the long bones: the experience at the Istituto Ortopedico Rizzoli. Am J Surg Pathol 1981;6:533–542.
85 Hales MS, Ferell LD: Fine-needle aspiration biopsy of tibial adamantinoma: a case report. Diagn Cytopathol 1988;4:67–70.
86 Lauricia R, Mody D, Macleay L, Kearns RJ, Ramzay I: Adamantinoma: a case report with aspiration cytology and differential diagnostic and immunohistochemical considerations. Acta Cytol 1992;36:951–956.
87 Gianelli U, Patriarca C, Moro A, Ponzoni M, Giardini R, Massimo M, Alfano RM, Armiraglio E, Nucifora P, Bosari S, Coggi G, Parafioroti A: Lymphomas of the bone: a pathological an clinical study of 54 cases. Int J Surg Pathol 2002;10:257–266.
88 Nagasaka T, Nakamura S, Medeiros LJ, Juco J, Lai R: Anaplastic large cell lymphoma presented as bone lesions: a clinicopathologic study of six cases and review of the literature. Mod Pathol 2000;13:1143–1149.
89 Bakshi NA, Ross CW, Finn WG, Valdez R, Ruiz R, Koujok K, Schnitzer B: Alk-positive anaplastic large cell lymphoma with primary bone involvement in children. Am J Clin Pathol 2006;125:57–63.
90 Ostrowski ML, Inwarsa CY, Strickler JG, Witzig TE, Wenger DE, Unni KK: Osseous Hodgkin disease. Cancer 1999;85:1166–1178.
91 Lin F, Staerkel G, Fanning CV: Cytodiagnosis of primary lymphoma of bone on fine-needle aspiration cytology specimens: review of 25 cases. Diagn Cytopathol 2003;28:205–211.
92 Söderlund V, Skoog L, Tani E, Bauer HGF, Kreicbergs A: Diagnosis of skeletal lymphoma and myeloma by radiology and fine-needle aspiration cytology. Cytopathology 2001;12:157–167.
93 Ozdemirli M, Fanburg-Smith JC, Hartmann DP, Shad AT, Lage JM, Magrath IT, Azumi N, Harris NL, Cossman J, Jaffe ES: Precursor B-lymphoblastic lymphoma presenting as a solitary bone tumor and mimicking Ewing's sarcoma: a report of four cases and review of the literature. Am J Surg Pathol 1998;22:795–804.
94 Akhtar M, Ali MA, Bakry M, Sackey K, Sabbah R: Fine-needle aspiration biopsy of Langerhans histiocytosis (histiocytosis X). Diagn Cytopathol 1993;9:527–533.
95 Shabb N, Fanning CH, Carrasco C: Diagnosis of eosinophilic granuloma by fine needle aspiration with concurrent institution of therapy. Diagn Cytopathol 1993;9:3–12.
96 Pohar-Marinsek Z, Us-Krasovec M: Cytomorphology of Langerhans cell histiocytosis. Acta Cytol 1996;40:1257–1264.
97 Kilpatrick SE: Fine needle aspiration biopsy of Langerhans cell histiocytosis: are ancillary studies necessary for a 'definitive diagnosis'? Acta Cytol 1998;42:820–823.
98 Shih LY, Chen TH, Lo WH: Skeletal metastasis from occult carcinoma. J Surg Oncol 1992;51: 109–113.
99 Katagiri H, Takahashi M, Inagaki J, Sugiura H, Ito S, Iwata H: Determining the site of the primary cancer in patients with skeletal metastasis of unknown origin: a retrospective study. Cancer 1999;86:533–537.
100 Saad RS, Clary KM, Liu Y, Silverman JF, Raab SS: Fine needle aspiration biopsy of vertebral lesions. Acta Cytol 2004;48:39–46.
101 Akhtar I, Flowers R, Siddiqi A, Heard K, Baliga M: Fine needle aspiration biopsy of vertebral and paravertebral lesions: retrospective study of 124 cases. Acta Cytol 2006;50:364–371.

Index